Group

Voices Within the Journey of
Eating Disorder Recovery

Karen :
May you have peace within your
Mind, Body, and Heart

By Annette Aberdale-Kendra

RN BSN CCAP

Annette Aberdale-Kendra

Mt. Holyoke College 2013

Dear First Edition Reader,

Thank you for looking at my book.

This place in the book is where you usually find praiseful words from famous people . . . but I don't know any famous people, and anyway, this is not a book of, by, or for famous people. The simple fact that you have picked my book up and are reading these words means that you are exactly the kind of person whose praiseful words – or constructively critical words, I admit – could be most helpful to other readers of a second edition.

So if you read this book, and find it useful (or find ways that you think I could make it more useful) I would like to hear from you. You will find my email address on the copyright page.

I also would like to have a page or two of readers' thoughts for this book's next edition. Please let me know if you like my book, and a few words about why. For a first-time author, and one who's not primarily a writer, putting these thoughts out into the world with black ink on white paper is daunting, and your thoughts about my work are precious to me.

Again, thank you.

Annette

Group

Voices Within the Journey of Eating Disorder Recovery

By Annette Aberdale-Kendra

RN BSN CCAP

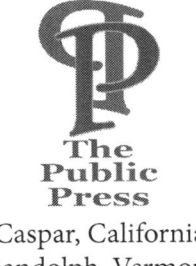

The
Public
Press

Caspar, California
Randolph, Vermont

cover concept: Annette Aberdale-Kendra
cover design: Michael Potts
book design: Michael Potts

Contents

About the Author

Annette Aberdale-Kendra RN BSN CCAP is a practicing nurse in Western Massachusetts. She offers a perspective that combines her interest and expertise in mental, physical, and spiritual health. She has been involved in a variety of community based initiatives to increase awareness, support, and education regarding eating disorders, healthy body image, and media literacy. As part of this effort, Annette has developed and facilitated numerous Psycho-Educational groups for young women with eating disorders. Furthermore, she has assisted a professional team in the development of a mentoring program for girls in early recovery.

Annette has addressed many school and public communities providing workshops to students, faculty, parents, and other individuals. In addition to these contributions, Annette is a Certified Clinical Aromatherapist and the founder of Balanced You Clinical Aromatherapy for Women. She assists women of all ages in achieving optimal health and well being on a mental, physical, and spiritual level. Annette lives in Western Massachusetts with her husband and two sons.

Acknowledgements

My two sweet boys Collin and Nicholas, thank you for constantly reminding me of all the beauty in "this moment". You are both my little teachers. It is to you that I dedicate this book.

Rich, you believe in my dreams and encourage my uniqueness – thank you for embracing my soul.

Mom and dad, your love has held me up. Thank you for your constant support.

The Journey

One day you finally knew
what you had to do, and began,
though the voices around you
kept shouting
their bad advice --
though the whole house
began to tremble
and you felt the old tug
at your ankles.
"Mend my life!"
each voice cried.
But you didn't stop.
You knew what you had to do,
though the wind pried
with its stiff fingers
at the very foundations,
though their melancholy
was terrible.
It was already late
enough, and a wild night,
and the road full of fallen
branches and stones.
But little by little,
as you left their voices behind,
the stars began to burn
through the sheets of clouds,
and there was a new voice
which you slowly
recognized as your own,
that kept you company
as you strode deeper and deeper
into the world,
determined to do
the only thing you could do --
determined to save
the only life you could save.

– Mary Oliver

Introduction

Since I began my work with young women several years ago, I have had a concern about the increasing number of girls and women who are developing eating disorders and body image issues worldwide. I have been aware that the region I live in and work, Western Massachusetts, has reflected this disturbing trend. I have also been aware that although the number of cases of eating disorders continues to rise, there is a significant shortage of therapy groups for girls and women with this problem.

As a clinical person in the healing profession, I truly understand the deficit this creates. From my previous experience working with young women, I understand that this forum of support can provide individuals in physical or emotional distress an opportunity to be heard by others who share a similar experience. I believe that this kind of involvement offers invaluable comfort, validation, education, and new perspectives, which facilitate growth and healing. I am well aware that current research in the field repeatedly and clearly supports the use of group therapy as an adjunct to individual therapy in treating eating disorders. This is why I have created and offered therapy groups to many young women with eating disorders.

My intent is to bring this group forum – which has been such a necessary, effective, and helpful resource – to a much larger audience to make more available that which has been unavailable or, at best, scarce. I have decided there is no better way to do this than to format an actual book as if it were a nine week psycho-educational group.

In designing this book, I have made some deliberate choices about the nature of the text, which I believe sets it apart from other eating disorder books. I do not want to offer a self-help book on eating disorders, written with the intent of being inspirational, that could then later be misconstrued and become triggering. Clearly, this is challenging, because when people are very entrenched in a disorder that can be addictive in nature, as eating

Group: Voices Within the Journey of Eating Disorder Recovery

disorders are, just about any mention of unhealthy behaviors can be triggering. You can end up reinforcing exactly what you are trying to discourage. I realize this is never the deliberate intent of the author; however, many girls who are ambivalent about recovery, which many are, purchase eating disorder material or go onto descriptive eating disorder websites and, as a result, end up reinforcing unhealthy behaviors. To minimize the chances of this occurrence, I have decided to make the text of this book specifically recovery focused. I am very careful to avoid extensive conversation about graphic eating disorder behaviors and not allow discussion about weight and size. I devote my attention to what is behind the eating disorder behavior – how it develops and how individual characteristics and life circumstances can impact behaviors – rather than focusing on just behaviors themselves.

Certain themes have emerged from the increasing amount of information and research available on the subject of eating disorders over the last ten years that suggests that although no two experiences are alike, there are commonalities amongst people with eating disorders. I am calling these common features **the core issues**. In my experience, it can be very helpful to develop an understanding of these issues when facing recovery. Therefore, I will discuss the core issues as each Week begins and then they will be further explored through the experiences of each group member. In learning about the core issues in this way, it is my intention to make it easier to have a deeper understanding about these issues and how they can impact behaviors and eventual recovery.

The book is set up to capture a group of five young girls meeting together for nine consecutive weeks. Each Week has a new topic, and there is discussion related to these specific core issues. The core issues appear woven into the Weeks. They appear as follows: Week One: Feelings, Week Two: The Voice of the Eating Disorder, Week Three: Perfectionism, Week Four: Fear, Week Five: Control, Week Six: One Woman's Recovery, Week Seven: Hungers, Week Eight: Culture and Values. The Ninth Week: Moving Forward, is primarily devoted to saying goodbye, as the girls explore the challenge of change as they move forward in their recovery.

Within each group, there is an opportunity to look at these core challenges through the eyes of the participants. From the dialogue between the girls and Jillian, the facilitator, it is easy to learn about the deep emotional needs of these young women and their personal, familial, and developmental challenges. Within each group the facilitator presents specific coping strategies to assist the group in being better able to deal with these challenges. At the end of each group/week, before departing, Jillian offers the girls *Words of Hope* so each session is closing on a note of encouragement and inspiration.

In the final chapter of the book, Coming Back Together, the girls and Jillian reconnect after their long Summer break. She invites them to attend a reunion to gather strength and discuss how they fared with the challenges in their lives and the success or not of their newly acquired skills. From within this context, they tell of their Summer adventures, their challenges, and their triumphs. Finally, in closing, a great amount of emotion and strength is demonstrated as the group comes to a final end.

As I write this book, I realize my focus is young women with eating disorders ages sixteen to twenty-two, primarily because this is the age group I have worked with. However, I consistently am learning that no matter what age, whether there is a diagnosis of Bulimia, Anorexia, Binge-eating disorder, or a struggle with body image issues, many females share similar challenges. Many use food as a way to calm their emotional and spiritual hungers. Others may try to shrink their bodies into a size they think will make them feel worthy and valued. While still others spend their lives apologizing for the bodies they have, living their lives from one diet to the next. My intention is for this book to be for women of all backgrounds and cultures.

In providing Psychoeducational groups for young women with eating disorders and body image issues, I have learned invaluable lessons. I have been constantly reminded of the strength, resiliency, and generosity of the human spirit. These groups reinforced my understanding of the complexity of eating disorders and their numerous causative factors: biological, psychological, and environmental. I do believe that in order to treat them most effectively, requires a multidimensional approach – one which will address the mental, physical, emotional, and spiritual aspects of the disorder. Most importantly, I have discovered that by providing a forum in which women can commune regularly, to share with each oither their deepest joys and sorrows, has proven to assist them profoundly in the process of healing. And it has been through being witness to the power of these exchanges that I am further inspired.

This book is meant to be an affirming guide. I want it to offer comfort and validation from within its pages. My words are intended to be an antidote to the many harsh and critical messages so many young women encounter in their lives. My intention is not only to reach those struggling with an eating disorder, but also the parents, friends, loved ones, and therapists who are supporting the recovery process of others. Please join myself and five amazing young women. Witness the group unfold, as we travel together through this journey of eating disorder recovery.

Author's Note

The young women in **Group: Voices Within the Journey of Eating Disorder Recovery** are fictionalized characters. I have invited these young women to participate in this therapy group, to share with one another their journey of recovery, because I want many young women to have the opportunity to benefit from a group experience. I want so many others to have the same chance to feel understood and supported while experiencing and learning about the process of recovery. I have based the experiences and challenges of these young women on several years of listening to girls both within my professional work and within my personal life. They are composites of the many remarkable young women who entrusted me with their stories, and I have been careful not to reveal their true identities.

Although this book is meant to be a support during times of challenge, I do not recognize it to be the only means of support. If you have an eating disorder or you are struggling with food or weight concerns, I highly recommend you use this book in conjunction with other forms of therapy. The most effective approach for treating eating disorders is to create a multidisciplinary team which consists of the following practitioners: a physician who understands the potential medical complications of eating disorders, a therapist who is knowledgeable of the field, a nutritionist who understands the nuances of eating disorders, and a psychiatrist, if medication is warranted.

As you begin this journey, you may want to play with the idea of considering yourself as the sixth member of this group. Although you are reading about these young women and not actually meeting them, you may recognize similarities between their situations and yours, and this can be very powerful. Remember, this is your process, use this book as a tool to add ease and comfort to your own recovery. Come back to various weeks as you may need, when you are struggling with different issues. Use the stories that are about to unfold of these five women as guides for your own personal journey through eating disorder recovery.

Week One

Feelings

Throughout my experiences as a nurse, I have been constantly reminded that **feelings** are so important and central to our experience and existence as human beings. Feelings are basically an emotional gauge that we carry that helps us navigate our experiences. For some people this gauge can be more difficult to manage than it is for others.

In working with young women struggling with Anorexia, Bulimia, or Binge-eating disorder, it is clear that the issue of feelings can be very challenging during recovery. One reason for this is because when someone is struggling with an eating disorder, their personal emotional gauge may not be registering correctly. It either over reacts or under reacts. This then creates an imbalance where their feelings become too threatening to experience. When this happens, a person with an eating disorder will utilize unhealthy behaviors such as bingeing, purging, or restricting to try and regulate their experience and manage their feelings.

Many of the young women in the groups I have facilitated explain that they are truly afraid of their feelings and want to avoid them completely. They realize that because their emotional gauge is malfunctioning, it contributes to their unhealthy eating disorder behaviors and their need to keep doing them. This they believe will keep them safe. In other words, it becomes easier to focus on their body and food then face their feelings.

Many of the young women struggling with eating disorders oftentimes do not have positive role models to demonstrate ways of managing feelings in a healthy way. We live in an addictive culture that relies on many things to regulate emotions. In addition, today's society encourages a fast paced lifestyle, inhibiting time to relax and process our emotions, which ultimately leads to imbalance and feelings of anxiety.

As many begin recovery, they develop the skill of beginning to think about their needs and desires. This can be seen as taking an emotional inventory. Soon they are able to recognize when they "feel fat or ugly", it is necessary to pause and look inward to discover what they truly need.

Managing Feelings

One of the most effective ways to become more aware of and comfortable with feelings is **journaling**. Journaling can take many different forms. For many young women this can help regulate their own emotional gauges, while helping to decrease the imbalance of over reacting or under reacting. I encourage journaling to many of my group clients.

Journaling initiates a dialogue with oneself. It becomes a vehicle to go inward and allows the person to listen and connect with what they may be experiencing. They are able to safely express their thoughts and feelings as their process of recovery evolves and changes. I have found that when clients use this coping skill, it is an effective way for them to focus on what is behind their eating disorder behaviors.

As you read this Week, begin to notice how your own personal emotional gauge is registering. It is important to remember that one day it will be possible for your feelings to be felt and managed in a way that is safer and less threatening. You may want to begin experimenting with journaling. However you are becoming reacquainted with your feelings, allow the experiences of the group members to assist you in learning about your full range of emotions and the needs that exist alongside them.

Sometimes I don't want to be inside my body because I don't know what to do with all the feelings... It's as if I feel too much

– Carly

The girls enter the room for the first time and sit down in the chairs. Each of them exhibits some anxiety and uncertainty.

Jillian: I would like to welcome all of you here this evening. I am truly grateful to be facilitating this group. I realize coming here may not have been very easy for some of you and I feel great admiration and respect for each and every one of you.

As we begin our first group, I would like to take some time for us to become familiar with the space we will be joining each other in each week. This is the room we will be meeting in for the next eight weeks on Tuesday evenings. I have put the chairs in a circle for all of us to sit with pillows on the floor if you would be more comfortable. There are some blankets in the basket by the white door you came in from if anyone feels cold. This winter has been extremely cold, and on a snowy night like tonight, a blanket can be very comforting. I like to keep the blinds on the windows slightly opened. Right now it is dark outside, but in a few weeks the sun will still be shining at the time we meet. We are on the second floor so please know that nobody can see in this room very well from the outside. I also do not like bright artificial light, so I tend to keep the lights dim – if this is problem for any of you please tell me. Also, let me know if there is anything else any of you may need to feel more comfortable during our time together.

I would like to now share some of myself with all of you. Then each of you will have the opportunity to share as much or as little as you would like. The only requirement is I would like each of you to try to acknowledge one characteristic of yourself that you admire or accept. So, let's begin.

My name is Jillian. I have been a Registered Nurse for 15

years. I have enjoyed working with young women struggling with eating disorders and body image issues – I think mostly because as I was growing up I realized that many of the women in my life were unhappy with their bodies and external appearances. As I matured I wanted to reach out to women and empower them into feeling comfortable in their natural skin. I feel there is great power and opportunity for growth when females come together like we are this evening. My own personal interests include biking, painting, yoga, and meditation. I also enjoy being outdoors as often as I can and have recently taken up the hobby of bird watching. I actually have two characteristics that I have come to admire about myself. The first is the love and respect I feel for nature. The second characteristic is my light brown curly hair – I feel it suits my personality in many ways.

Now that I have shared about myself, I am wondering if there is anyone who may feel comfortable enough to tell about themselves.

Anika: I guess I can start.

I'm Anika and I'm twenty two. I live in Belchertown with my family. We moved to Massachusetts about sixteen years ago from a village in Eastern India to be closer to our family who moved here to America. All my aunts and uncles live in my same neighborhood, and we own a restaurant together. Oh, and I go to Holyoke Community College and am working on a degree in Business Administration. I've never been in a group before, so I'm very nervous, and I am not really sure what to expect. I am here, primarily, because my aunt told my mother she thinks it could help me control my weight – and then my family would be less ashamed of me. Right now, they don't think I'll ever be able to get married. I think I have been on every diet that exists and I feel so discouraged and ashamed with my body and my life. It is really hard for me to think of something I admire or accept about myself. The only good thing right now for me is I have a 4.0 average in school – and I really enjoy my classes this semester.

Jillian: Anika, it is very brave of you to begin. It is wonderful that you were able to offer yourself praise for your achievements with your education. You show great strength in challenging yourself.

Who feels that they could share next?

Taylor: I guess I will because I am sitting next to Anika and it feels like I am supposed to.

Jillian: You do not have to if you are not comfortable.

Taylor is looking down at her legs, crossing and uncrossing them, while pressing her fingers into them.

Taylor: It doesn't matter – my mother practically dragged me here anyway. So here goes nothing!

I'm Taylor and I'm from Turners Falls. Sad, I really don't know what to say, but I've been in a lot of groups before. I don't know if I will be able to come every week – it all depends on whether or not I can get a ride.

Jillian: Taylor, excuse me, but I wonder if you are uncomfortable sitting in these chairs. I can see you are moving around a lot and your facial expressions appear like maybe something is disturbing you.

Taylor: You don't miss a thing. It's just that this damn chair makes my legs look extra fat!

Jillian: Would you feel more comfortable sitting on a pillow on the floor? This would be fine if it helps you right now.

Taylor: Maybe later if I don't stop feeling so gross.

Anyway, I'm a junior in high school and my stupid guidance counselor told my mother about this group, and she thinks it would be good for me. So here I am! As far as what I admire about myself – that's easy – my yellow-green eyes. Many people have told me they are very seductive. Without these eyes I would be nothing.

Jillian: Taylor, you were very honest and that is admirable.

Please try to make yourself as comfortable as you can as we continue.

Taylor: I will.

You know – you seem pretty nice for someone who runs a group.

Jillian: I appreciate your kind words, Taylor.

Who would like to go next?

Carly: Hi, I'm Carly! I'm glad to meet all of you. It feels so warm in here.

Before I start to talk about myself I have to say I really love the golden yellow walls of this room. It reminds me of a Summer sunset. It just feels so warm and comfortable.

Jillian: It is nice to hear you feel so comfortable in this room.

Would you like to continue?

Carly: I am seventeen and I go to school at Northfield Mount Herman, but I am originally from outside of Boston. My mom runs a day care out of our home. My sister and I were in it when we were young – it was the best! My dad manages a consulting business close to our home. I really love my family and I hate that they are so concerned about me. I'm kind of stressed out about being here right now because I am in the middle of some big exams and I really should be studying. I'm also about to take the SATs and beginning to look at colleges. I'm not sure how all of this is going to work out. I have had an eating disorder for a long time, and sometimes fall back into old patterns, but I don't see why everyone is so concerned. I'm told if I don't get my weight up I won't be able to swim on the team this season. But if they really stopped to look, they would see that just about every girl in the dorm has some kind of eating issue.

Taylor, I want to tell you, your legs are so thin and muscular. I don't see an ounce of fat on them. I mean I play one or two sports every season and I wish my legs looked like yours.

Taylor: Trust me – it is just what I am wearing.

Jillian: Carly, I wonder how it feels for you listening to Taylor discussing her difficult thoughts about her body?

Carly: I don't know. I guess I feel like she has a great body. If she had my body, then she could complain.

Jillian: That sounds very difficult to sit with.

I would like all of you girls to know that when you are struggling with an eating disorder or body image issues, talk like this may become triggering and difficult for you to hear. I want to assure you that we will discuss these issues as I review the guidelines for this group and I hope it will make this topic of triggering less upsetting for each of you.

Taylor: You know another thing I am good at, messing things up. Here I go again, just like my parents say.

See, this group crap isn't for me, no matter how many I have been in.

Jillian: Taylor, you do belong here with us and you are doing fine. You have done nothing wrong. We are just beginning to learn about each other and none of us know what to expect. I believe that your presence in this group is very important.

Taylor: We'll see! Whatever – sorry to interrupt.

Jillian: No need for apologizing.

If we can, I would like to give Carly the opportunity to continue.

Carly: All I have left to say is something I like about myself.

The one thing that I have always enjoyed is singing and acting. I feel like I can become anybody and be anything. I mean it's the best, because it allows me to step out of who I am and become somebody else. I love it!

Jillian: Carly, thank you for sharing something that is so important to you. It is wonderful that you have a talent that you feel so deeply for.

Who would like to continue?

Min gazes down as she begins talking in a very soft voice.

Min: Hello, I'm Min. I am from Seoul, but I live at my school, Suffield Academy.

Anika: Where are you from? I cannot hear you very well.

Min: I'm from Seoul, Korea, and I am sorry to be talking so quietly, I just feel very nervous.

Jillian: Min, it is very natural to feel nervous and uncomfortable beginning a group like this. As we continue to come together and learn more about ourselves and each other, the anxiety that each of you may feel about being here will become less. Would it be okay for you to continue telling us about yourself?

Min: Sure. I will try to speak louder and if anyone cannot hear me please let me know.

Jillian: Min, begin again when you are ready.

Min: I am a freshman at Suffield Academy. It has been very difficult for me being so far away from home while trying to keep up on my studies and become familiar with the ways of the American Culture. I've never been in a group either. I'm hoping I can learn more about how to control my weight because my family said I am eating too much and I am gaining weight. My best friend at home said I'm probably just getting used to eating differently while I'm away at school and not to worry so much about it. I didn't even really notice it was a problem until other people said something. Now, it's hard to stop thinking about it. I feel so self conscious. Recently, my roommate told someone at school I was throwing up in the bathroom, and the school told me if I continued they might have to send me home on medical leave. I never expected any of this to happen. I guess I am kind of scared. I have to apologize, but right now I cannot honestly think of one thing I admire about myself. I'm sorry.

Jillian: Min, it is important to recognize that you have shared what you feel you could here tonight with us and I hope this group will offer you the insight you are searching for.

I would like to take this opportunity to remind all of you that there may be moments during these groups that may be difficult for you to participate in. There is no pressure or judgment here. My hope for each of you is that you are able to come here each week and be in each moment in the ways that you are comfortable – challenging yourself only when you feel you can. Each one of you wonderful young women has a place in this group and it is important that you take what you need from our time together.

Stephanie, it can be your time now to introduce yourself.

Stephanie: I will talk about me, but I want to tell you, Min, I think your wire-rim glasses are beautiful. When you walked in the room, I noticed them. Then after hearing you speak, their beauty really matches your personality.

Min: Thank you very much, Stephanie. I don't know what to say.

Stephanie: Nothing needs to be said.

Hi everyone, I'm Stephanie and I am a junior at the University of Massachusetts. I've had my eating disorder for a long time, and I've been seeing a therapist who thinks a group could be really good for me. She's been trying to find one for a long time, but there just aren't any around. Last week she saw a flier about this one, so I thought I would give it a try. I apologize for the way I keep clearing my throat – it's kind of a nervous habit I guess. Anyway, I don't really know what to expect either. I feel sort of bad being here, because I feel like my mother needs me at home. As for what I admire about myself, what comes to my mind is how I enjoy helping others. It's when I feel the happiest.

Jillian: Stephanie thank you for allowing us to learn about you.

I realize being in a group is a new experience for some of you and may be very uncomfortable. Most people are not used to being asked to share some of their most personal thoughts and feelings publicly. I ask that you try to challenge yourselves by practicing to become more comfortable with this uneasiness. As I said before, it should get easier. However, having said that, I will also support you if you are unable to confront certain topics, either as part of the group or individually. What makes discussion about eating disorders that much more difficult is people tend to carry so much shame with them. Women who have Anorexia, Bulimia, Binge-eating disorder, or a combination thereof often feel they must protect themselves from the harsh judgment of others or from being misunderstood. As each of you become more familiar with all of us in the group and you realize you share many commonalities, you should begin feeling more at ease.

Before I continue on about the group is there anything anybody would like to say?

Carly examines the room, particularly
in the direction of the window.

Carly: Jillian, as we are all talking I keep noticing that rock candle on top of the bookshelf by the window. I have never seen anything like that. Is it some special type of candle?

Jillian: That is a salt crystal candle holder. The heat from the flame allows the salt crystal to purify the air with negative ions. I will be lighting it every time we meet. Salt crystals can be very healing and therapeutic.

Carly, it is nice to see that you are comfortable enough to inquire about the surroundings we are coming together in.

Carly: Thanks for the explanation.

I want to ask my parents to get one of those for our home!

Jillian: Enjoy it.

Does anybody else have any questions or concerns?

Stephanie: I apologize. I know this is probably a really inappropriate time to ask this, but if I don't I will be distracted by my curiosity.

Is that your old fashioned roll top desk Jillian? It is so beautiful. It reminds me of the one my grandmother had at her house – except hers was a much lighter wood. I would play school with it all the time when I was younger.

Jillian: It sounds like the desk attracted you because it was something familiar to you. Let me explain about this desk.

It was my mother's when she was young. Her grandfather made it for her when she was six years old. I have always enjoyed wonderful antiques, and when I graduated from college my mother offered it to me. I have kept it in that same corner for many years here in my office. You all may see me getting papers from it now and then because I use it to store references and information I use for these groups. I am very glad you asked.

Stephanie: Now my curiosity is not controlling my thoughts.

Jillian: If there are not any other questions about this room, I would like to discuss some of the expectations I have of the group.

Our group will begin each Tuesday at six o'clock in the evening. Please try and arrive as close to six as possible so we can begin on time. I find sometimes one and a half hours can go by very quickly. Also, please make every effort to attend each group. I realize you all have busy, full lives but in order to be an effective group, each of us needs to be here consistently. If you cannot attend, please call me prior to the group time so I can let the rest of the group know you will not be coming that evening. Next, it is important for all of us to show respect for each other when speaking. Another expectation that I hope will be comforting for everyone, as I mentioned earlier, is when we come together as a group, I would like to ask that we refrain from any discussion that revolves around numbers like weight, calories, amounts, clothing size, etc. This type of talk can become triggering and disturbing to our cohesive group. Finally, if an issue arises that any of you girls feel uncomfortable about – please speak up during the group time or see me before or after the group. The intention is for all of you to feel safe and comfortable here.

Are there any concerns or comments?

Anika: I feel so relieved!

As I sat here listening I began to feel so overwhelmed thinking we were going to be discussing diets, exercise habits, binge/purge cycles, etc. Now I feel slightly more comfortable with the idea of me being in a group like this. I am looking forward to learning more about how this whole group process works for girls struggling like we are.

Jillian: Let me spend some time talking a little about why I feel therapeutic groups are so valuable for people with eating disorders.

The concept of engaging people in groups to promote healing and well being is not a new one. In one form or another, groups have been around for some sixty years. Long ago, they were not called therapy groups; they were encounter groups or T-groups, and their overall focus was not the same as it is now. These were more human relation and training groups. However, many have long since known that when you gather together a group of people who share a similar problem and they are able to communicate to one another about their challenges, they grow and change in significant ways. Take, for instance, groups for people with cancer. Studies have shown repeatedly that through the process of sharing, patients feel less isolated, more understood, increase their knowledge about diagnosis and treatment, and may actually go on to live longer and happier lives.

In the research-based book called ***Group Therapy with Cancer Patients*** by David Spiegel, M.D. and Katherine Classen, Ph.D this idea is further supported and explained.

I will read a piece of this to you.

> It is clear from this research that expression of relevant emotions and direct discussions of difficult subject matters enhances rather than hinders quality of life and may actually increase survival time of women with breast cancer. The group experience offers to these patients a place in which they belong because of rather

than despite, their illness. Furthermore it constitutes a place where they can express feelings that may upset them and their loved ones.

I realize this is a lot of information, but it can be beneficial to have an understanding of the effectiveness groups can have. In fact, equally valuable are recovery groups such as Alcoholics Anonymous or Narcotics Anonymous. The structure and support of these groups help people to transform unhealthy behaviors and learn new strategies for coping. Within these settings, members feel they are no longer alone, and it is through compassion and acceptance of these communities that they find the support necessary to change.

Does anybody have any questions or concerns related to what I have talked about up to now?

Stephanie: I have a quick question. What are we going to talk about each week? Is this going to be the focus or do we just go around the circle like we did tonight talking about our own experiences?

Jillian: A very appropriate question, Stephanie.

Let me take a moment to explain in a little more detail, so you all will know a bit more of what to expect each week.

For the next several weeks, we will come together and discuss many of the struggles and triumphs that each of you may encounter. We will begin each evening with a check in that allows each of you to discuss how things have been for you since the last time we were together. The group will then unfold as it may. Before we part at the end of each group I will read to you the *Words of Hope*. These are small thoughts that I have composed to remind each of you to be kind to yourself. I have a whole notebook full I have created over the years I have been working with young women struggling with eating disorders and/or body image issues. Based on what comes up during our time together each week, I will choose one that seems appropriate. It is an opportunity to end each week on an uplifting note of encouragement.

I would like everyone to know, Week Six we will not be following our usual group format. We will be having a guest speaker. From past experience, this works out very well. It is a little more than half way through our time together and I am certain some growth and change will have occurred up to that point for each of you. I believe it can be very valuable to hear the actual story of how one woman recovered from an eating disorder. If there will be any other changes occurring in the usual group format, we can discuss them as we move on.

Taylor: Damn, you really have an interesting way of doing a group. I've been in a few groups before, but they have never been anything like this.

Jillian: That is a nice compliment, Taylor. I truly hope all of you find this group style to be comfortable and beneficial.

Because this is our first evening together, I like to pick a topic to begin discussing, just to help "break the ice" as we begin our group process. So this evening I decided I would like to take a few minutes and look at the role feelings play in each of your lives, with your eating disorder, and within recovery. I have decided to start here because for so many, this is such a difficult area – one that reaches into every aspect of life and one that so strongly correlates with behaviors either with or without an eating disorder. I am sure we all are experiencing many different feelings here this evening. Let me explain more.

As human beings, we are given the unique capacity to experience a myriad of emotions at any point in time. With the body as our medium, we can feel sadness by tightening in our throats, happiness through our spontaneous laughter, embarrassment from the flush in our cheeks, and fear through our racing hearts. For most of us, these physical sensations function as a useful gauge – a barometer which assists us in measuring when it is better to back away from a situation or when to move in closer. These physical cues tell us when our body needs rest, when we are hungry, when we should seek solace in the support of a loved one and when to be alone. These feelings provide us with vital information to help us determine how we should act and behave.

Because the capacity to feel is such an integral part of the human experience, most of us cannot avoid times in our lives when we may be overwhelmed by the magnitude of their impact. For instance, it is not unusual for us to be overcome by emotion when we have achieved noteworthy recognition or praise for our accomplishments. It is also quite typical for us to be overcome with joy when we learn someone we admire feels the same way about us. And just as significant events in our lives can bring upon overwhelming happiness, so too can they engulf us in despair. Both extremes of emotion can cause us to feel a temporary disequilibrium or imbalance, but for the most part, we can find our way through these tumultuous squalls. We ride them out until we have achieved a state of normalcy and balance. There are times, however, when we need the temporary assistance of another to help us find our way. During these times, it is helpful to seek out support of a minister, counselor, friend, or loved one – someone to accompany us as we are consoled by the passing of time.

Min: I'm so sorry to interrupt.

I understand what you are saying, but it's hard for me to see how feelings play a role in eating disorders.

Jillian: No apologies are needed. Ask questions whenever you need to.

Let me explain.

I have found that women who have eating disorders do not have this same emotional elasticity to help them return to a balanced state. Within the therapy groups I have facilitated, many young women with Anorexia and Bulimia have stated they have a much harder time navigating the ever changing emotional terrain that comes with being human. For many of them, the disequilibrium they experience is not temporary, and it is often so overwhelming it causes them to resort to unhealthy ways of coping. Many have expressed to me that when they feel sadness, joy, or anger, they are so overcome by the depths of their emotion that they become completely engulfed and swept away. They feel so out of control by the magnitude of these storms that they, in turn, will over-focus on food and weight so they can escape the other parts of life causing them despair.

Other group members have described a slightly different experience, but one that also reflects their extreme challenge with emotion. These young women describe feeling disconnected from any sensations in their bodies, unaware of how their body might be responding at any given time. They feel numb to the typical fluctuations in mood, and when they do feel emotion, it is only in reaction to what they experience about food and weight – not the normal day to day occurrences. For them, their eating disorder has become a protective (though unhealthy) barrier which insulates them from life.

Does this help clarify how eating disorders and feelings may relate?

Min: Yes, thank you.

So, what you are saying is many women with eating disorders may feel like a prisoner to their feelings and therefore try to control them?

Jillian: Well said. In 1999, Andrea Lobu and Marsea Marcus, two therapists who specialize in the treatment of eating disorders, published *The Don't Diet, Live-It Workbook*. Within their book, they explain the difficulty people with eating disorders have dealing with emotion. Let me share an excerpt from this book with all of you:

> Normally, feelings flow through us like clouds drifting in the sky. Sadness, joy, fear, and peace come and go in varying degrees at different speeds throughout our days. When we're on a road trip, we have to deal with and adjust our plans according to the weather. While we never think that we could actually control the weather, we most certainly try to control our feelings. Those of us with food and weight issues don't let our feelings drift by like clouds, simply noticing them, or perhaps commenting on their form and dimension. Instead, we try to construct walls to hold them back, or

we bury them deep inside, or we try to change them into something they are not.

This is a lot to take in. I wonder what is happening for everyone as this topic of feelings is being discussed.

Carly: It's kind of funny that we are talking about feelings because I was just talking to my roommate about this, and she thinks I am always creating drama in my life. But I really can't help it. Other people tell me I have mood swings – I am either high or low. I never really know how I am going to feel from one minute to the next, and the slightest little thing can pull me down.

Jillian: Carly, this is wonderful insight.

It sounds very challenging and scary to feel so consumed by feelings.

Carly: It is, but keeping up in my studies, sports, and theater seem to help me at times.

Taylor: That sounds a lot like me! I never feel like I have any damn control over my moods. It's like I'm always PMSing. I can be going along fine, and if someone at school makes a nasty comment about me or I don't like what I am wearing, forget about it – my whole day is ruined.

The other day I was getting ready for school, and I think I was arguing with my brother, and then I couldn't find anything to wear that looked right, so I didn't end up leaving my stupid bed for the whole morning. I was so miserable.

Jillian: Both of you girls have done a wonderful job sharing some of your personal experiences that demonstrate how strong and overwhelming feelings can be. It sounds like both of you are saying, in your own way, that your feelings carry with them a presence of being too powerful, that they have control over you and, as a result, they can make life feel out of control and unpredictable at times.

I have found that many girls with eating disorders experience a sensation of being flooded all at once with emotion. They feel overcome by this surge, often to the point where they are unable to recognize their individual feeling states. It is as if they are drowning in a sea of emotion. They cannot identify feelings of sadness, anger, fear, or frustration. They only know that they must do something to help them regain their ground in order to feel better.

It is also not unusual for women with this kind of extreme emotional sensitivity and reactivity to be unable to identify the situation or event that contributed to the reaction. What they are more than likely to do is feel responsible for a situation they can neither explain nor describe, and one they undoubtedly have nothing to do with. Oftentimes, this feeling of responsibility or shame translates into feeling of body hatred and self loathing.

It is difficult to realize that when you are caught in the midst of a storm of blinding emotion, there are reasons and precipitants that have led to you being there. When this happens, it can be extremely helpful to realize you have needs behind these emotions, and it is often these undetected or unaddressed needs that will lead to unhealthy behaviors.

Taylor, I wonder if you can try to think back a little more and try to remember what it felt like to be arguing with your brother.

Taylor: I don't know. We always argue. He's a selfish jerk and he never listens to me. He only cares about himself and his slutty girlfriend.

Jillian: Do you remember what you were arguing about?

Taylor: Yeah, he thought I was taking too long in the bathroom, and he needed to get in there. Meanwhile, he spends half of his stupid, useless life in there! It's like I don't even exist!

Taylor is visibly pinching her thighs.

Can I please sit on the floor? This chair and my thighs don't agree.

Jillian: Please make yourself comfortable.

Do you think you can try to find some more words to describe how this experience feels to you?

Taylor: Violent! I want to hurt him, but he's too big. I feel angry, invisible…like I don't count in this world.

Jillian: Taylor, you are doing great exploring this situation.

I wonder if there is anywhere in your body you are feeling this anger as you talk about what happened? Being able to discover where in our body we carry different feelings can help us manage the magnitude that these emotions can develop into.

Taylor: I feel pressure on my chest.

Jillian: Try to take some slow, deep breaths. Imagine these breaths breathing into the pressure you feel.

What do you think you may have needed at the time that you weren't getting from him?

Taylor: I guess respect.

Jillian: That is truly understandable. It must be pretty hard living in a situation where you don't feel validated.

Did you realize all of that was going on inside of you at the time?

Taylor: No, I thought my mood was only about my ugly clothing and my disgusting body.

Jillian: Although difficult, it can be extremely helpful to try to uncover what the needs are behind your thoughts, feelings, and actions. At one time or another, we disconnect from them because they're too painful, but then they find other ways to come out.

Taylor, I feel great respect for you in this moment. You have demonstrated great strength in reliving this difficult experience.

Taylor: Thanks, I guess.

Sorry for the dramatic picture of my life that resembles a crappy Lifetime Channel Movie.

Carly: I don't want to dominate the conversation here, but I think I feel too much. Sometimes I don't even want to be inside my own body because I don't know what to do with all my emotions. I watch the news and it makes me so angry about how our country treats other people, and then I want to do something about it, but what can just one person do? Oh, and when I want something to work out a certain way, like an exam or a swim meet or something, I can't ever stop thinking about it – and worrying.

The other thing is, it's really hard to know sometimes if you're thinking something or feeling it.

Jillian: You are not dominating anything. This is our group and it is important that you are choosing to speak up.

You bring some very important observations about yourself. Thanks for sharing them.

It is absolutely true, when someone is overcome by emotion, it is difficult to see clearly what is going on or to pinpoint an exact feeling state. In order to help unravel this, it can be helpful to ask yourself to review what just really happened, as Taylor just did so effectively. It can also be helpful to think of emotions as sensations experienced through your body. Emotions are clues that we need something to be different. Whereas, thoughts can be seen as ideas, beliefs, and judgments you hold. Our thoughts can carry us to past and future moments that have little to do with the present moment we are in.

I wonder how this explanation is for you?

Carly: It gives me a lot to think about that I have never realized before or even understood.

Jillian: It is important to recognize recovery and healing is a process that requires learning about ourselves on many levels. The most important thing I can say to all of you is to be gentle with yourselves when it comes to your feelings. As we discussed, feel in your body where you carry the feelings, breathe, and try to discover what you may need.

I wonder how everyone else in the group is doing as we are working through this very important topic of feelings?

Anika: Well, I guess for me, one of the most difficult things is to be alone, and maybe it's because it's so hard to feel things.

When you're alone, there aren't as many distractions. That's usually when I have my hardest time with food. I overeat. And then everyone gets mad at me because I eat everyone else's food. I feel so embarrassed. I don't even realize I'm doing it. Sometimes I have to go out and replace the food so they don't know it's missing.

Jillian: Anika, I wonder when you discovered that being or feeling alone is something that triggers your behaviors?

Anika: Probably about a year and a half ago when I began college.

Jillian: This is very important insight for you into understanding the role your eating disorder may have in your life. For many people, their eating disorder behaviors become a way of protecting themselves from some very painful or overwhelming emotions.

Anika: How could these eating behaviors be protecting me when, afterwards, I feel so ashamed and disgusting?

Jillian: This is an excellent point, Anika, and I hope as our weeks together evolve and we explore more about what is behind these eating disorder behaviors, this phenomenon will become clearer for all of you.

Anika: I am looking forward to this, because all of this talk and self learning is very new to me.

Stephanie: I don't mean to interrupt, but don't you think it's easier to just focus on the whole weight/body/food issue than to really look at what's going on? At least there is a familiarity or a sameness that goes along with it. I've done a lot of work around this with my individual therapist, and we both decided that, for me, it doesn't feel safe to feel my feelings. There are too many things that are just too scary to look at.

I think sometimes I don't even like thinking things are going well, because then I start to worry about when they're going to come crashing down.

Jillian: Stephanie, I believe what you are saying is, no matter how miserable you are with our eating disorder, there is consistency, a predictability that goes along with it, and with your life, you don't have that same element of control, and it's too overwhelming.

You bring up some really powerful insights and discoveries you've made, and it's clear you have done a lot of work around this.

I think it's important for all of you wonderful women in this room this evening to realize your eating disorder is there in your lives for an important reason. This journey of recovery is about learning why and how it plays the part in your lives it does and then finding the tools and support to begin making changes.

Are there any other thoughts any of you would like to add?

Alright then, as we continue on this evening, I would like all of you to know, I truly appreciate all the sharing that many of you have offered related to the topic of feelings. I am certain the topic of emotions and how they affect each of you will be a theme that will repeat itself in this group and within each of your recoveries. Because of this I would like to invite you all to keep a journal of some kind throughout this journey. It can help you become more connected with what you are feeling and how your emotions impact behaviors.

Journaling can be an overwhelming task. I do not want to add any extra work to your lives. So I have prepared a list of questions which can be used as a guide to help stimulate or organize your thoughts. I like to call this list of questions *My Daily Check-In.* Using something like this check-in can be a guide to help familiarize you with the process for turning inward to listen to your thoughts and feelings. Keep in mind that a journal does not have to be elaborate memoirs which will later be graded. My hope is that as the group moves along it will be stirring up different thoughts and feelings. Being able to write them down in between sessions will give you a place to hold them until we meet again. Let's take a minute and let me read to you all the list of questions I have compiled. Just listen and let them resonate within you. Use them day to day in ways that feel best for you.

I got mad today when...
I was bored today when...
I became anxious today when...
I was confused when...
I got annoyed when...
I felt badly about myself when...
I laughed when...
I felt proud when...
I was disappointed when...
I felt sad when...
Other feelings I have had...

I wonder how listening to these questions was for everyone?

Anika: It seemed kind of nice. As you were reading, I was thinking these are things I would want to know about someone I care about. I realize at times I don't really enjoy too much about myself. Yet, it makes sense that connecting with yourself using a method like this can be helpful in being healthy.

Jillian: Anika, it is encouraging that you have found some comfort in this journaling idea.

I would like all of you to be able to leave this week's group with the knowledge that it is possible to approach the whole topic of having feelings in a way other than what you are accustomed to. If we were to look back over the discussion we have had today, we would see the theme that kept coming up repeatedly for each of you was the notion that feelings are not safe. What I hope to have offered all of you is a new perspective, suggesting there are ways to approach emotions which are neither threatening nor destabilizing. By learning to observe your feelings – to identify them and discover what is behind them – you are approaching them with a new distance. You are assuming a stance of curiosity, and with this new stance, it is much harder to be swept off your feet by them. Watch them, observe them, and learn from them until they pass. They will pass.

Before we part for this evening, I encourage each and every one of you to praise yourselves for being here and doing this work. Be kind to yourselves. I would like to invite all of you to experience the *Words of Hope*, which I mentioned earlier in the group. Please use these words in ways that are most useful for you. Relax and take few breaths as I share this hopeful and encouraging thought.

As you move through recovery, you will learn to recognize your feelings as helpful allies that are always there for you. You will discover your emotions are there to help guide you and assist you in making decisions for yourself. As you become healthier, you will find ways to be able to listen to them without having to fear them or run from them. You will find comfort in their warm embrace.

I wish you all a comfortable week. I look forward to seeing you next Tuesday.

Week Two

Voice of the Eating Disorder

In working with young women within eating disorder groups, I have found a commonality that I refer to as **the voice of the eating disorder**. I use this term to describe the constant bombardment by an inner voice that fills them with negative messages. It seems this negative self talk stems from anxiety that is often times present for these girls.

How does this inner voice develop? Well, many believe this inner negative voice develops out of low self esteem, overly critical parents, neglect, or abuse. There is also a cultural standard of perfectionism and flawlessness related to external appearance that impacts many young women's inner voices.

Let me describe this further. This is not an actual voice talking to these young women. All of us have internal dialogues occurring within our thoughts constantly that can be positive or negative. Yet when someone has an eating disorder, the negative dialogue forces the positive dialogue to almost completely disappear.

During recovery many girls begin a new struggle, one that includes this internal negative voice. This voice manages to keep them holding onto their eating disorder by offering them dysfunctional positive messages that temporarily help lift them up emotionally. For someone who is struggling with their feelings, this can be strangely comforting. Soon this internal dialogue changes without warning and usually begins to drag them into a place of greater anxiety and depression. It then appears despite the efforts of these young women to get ahead in life, this voice is always diminishing their self esteem. It is a truly self sabotaging voice.

Managing the Voice of the Eating Disorder

Within my nursing experience, I have found when counseling young women with eating disorders, **cognitive behavioral approaches** such as **affirmations** tend to be helpful for many. This new approach of coping helps the girls by retraining their thinking so they are not being barraged by so many negative thoughts. Affirmations create the ability to reprogram thoughts and therefore interrupt the negative banter. Cognitive behavioral approaches can also aide them in becoming aware of their thoughts while offering them a choice or sense of control over them.

When used consistently, affirmations allow positive dialogue to begin to develop and be heard again. Confronting the voice of the eating disorder in this way has allowed many young women the ability to discover new parts of themselves. This has proven to be very empowering for many during recovery from an eating disorder.

Have you ever noticed this negative self talk existing within yourself? Sometimes we are not even aware of its presence because we are so accustomed to it and consider it to be our norm. As you read this Week, believe that it is possible through recovery to be free from the ties of this negative inner banter. As your recovery evolves you may begin to look back and recognize how deceiving it truly was and realize the freedom you feel without being controlled by it. The thought of not obeying this voice may seem too overwhelming, but over time it is possible. You deserve to have the positive voice inside of you be heard again, and no longer succumbed by the voice of the disorder.

I try to give myself positive messages, but it's like watching the news with its constant ticker tape of negative talk running across my brain. I always feel like I am in the middle of a battlefield.

– Taylor

Jillian: Welcome back!

I am happy to see all of you again. You have all been in my thoughts during this past week.

Carly is sitting in her chair in a fetal like position, holding her knees up to her chest.

Carly: Could I take a blanket. I have two sweaters on with my scarf and I am still cold. My coach and doctor keep telling me I feel cold so often because I've lost too much weight. I'm so tired of hearing this. It's winter, so it's cold! I'm not nearly as thin as some other girls on my swim team.

Taylor: Yeah, I hear what you are saying. My doctor has told me the same thing. Some stupid explanation like, "When you lose too much weight and body fat, your body is more sensitive to feeling cold." Whatever!

Jillian: That is correct, Taylor. Eating disorders can have many physiological effects on your bodies. Some of the most common problems are Dehydration, Electrolyte Imbalance, Cardiac Issues, Changes or Loss of Menstrual Cycle, and early onset of Osteoporosis.

Carly: I don't know what all the fuss about me and my weight is. I do not have any of these problems.

Jillian: Carly, it can be easy to compare yourself to others and judge your level of illness. Some of these physiological effects do not show up for many years though.

Try to remember, everybody's body is different and will react differently to the stress of an eating disorder.

Carly, you may take as many blankets as you need to feel warm and be comfortable.

Carly: Thank you.

Stephanie: This all sounds so scary.

Jillian: It definitely is scary. I am sure many of you have heard from somebody how eating disorders can affect your bodies in many ways.

Stephanie: I think it is crazy that we all know the dangers our eating disorders can have on ourselves, yet we do it anyway.

Jillian: It can seem confusing, yet it is typical of an illness that is addictive in nature. The "numbing" or escape that one may get from carrying out their eating disorder behaviors far outweighs the risks involved.

I think for this moment it is important that some of the physical issues have been addressed, yet I feel it is equally important to mention that it is not necessary to become overly consumed with what "can" occur. The human body is very resilient. I believe if the emotional status of a person improves and becomes healthier, the physical body will follow and do the same.

Stephanie: That is somewhat comforting.

Carly, would you like to sit over here where I am away from the window, it may feel warmer.

Carly: No, but I appreciate it!

Jillian: As we begin our second week together, does anyone have anything they would like to share about their week or the last group?

Carly: I'm sorry to talk again, but I have been doing a lot of thinking, and I'm feeling pretty discouraged.

I thought I was so done with this eating disorder, you know? Recovered! Now, here it is again, dictating my life – what I do, who I see, what I can't do – all over again!

Jillian: It must be very disappointing to realize it is more of a problem right now than you wanted to admit. You have struggled with it for a while.

I believe recovery from an eating disorder is an ongoing process, and there are different stages people go through, similar to recovery from any other kind of addiction. For most of us, the process is not a linear or clear-cut one. We may move back and forth depending on the challenges we're facing, the kind of support we're getting, and how much resolution there has been in the past. You may find you are in a much different place, both mentally and emotionally, than you were three years ago when you became so ill. Not all setbacks mean you are relapsing.

When you spoke, Carly, I heard great strength and determination along with frustration. This is a difficult process and it is important for all of you to be aware that recovery will have ups and downs.

It may be helpful if I take a moment to discuss the different stages of recovery. I hope this will help you, Carly, in fact all of you, to be patient with yourselves as you embark on this journey of change.

Within the recovery process, many theorists have studied addiction and examined how individuals move through different phases of change. As LoBue and Marcus suggest in their workbook that I mentioned last week, people move through four stages when recovering from an eating disorder: *Denial, Transition, Early Recovery and Ongoing Recovery.*

They explain that within the *Denial Stage* we are unable to see there is an emotional component to our eating disorder, and we have great difficulty looking to others for support. We may acknowledge there is a problem or we are unhappy with our lives, but we believe if we could eat less or control our eating we would be happier. During this stage, most people are unable to see clearly the true impact their eating disorder has on their lives and on those who care about them.

In the *Transition Stage*, we begin to see there are emotional problems that reach beyond the scope of our bingeing, purging, restricting, or critical perception of our bodies. We begin to acknowledge we have unresolved feelings and needs and we can see we lack the tools necessary to cope with them. During this stage, many people try to abstain from unhealthy behaviors with inadequate support and begin to feel overcome by the emotions they were unable to manage before. Therefore, this is a time when having adequate outside support is essential. During this stage, we begin to identify the situations and circumstances that propel us toward an episode of self-loathing and unhealthy eating, and there is motivation to take a healthier path.

Within *Early Recovery*, we have a deepened understanding of ourselves, our emotions, and the potential pitfall that could send us in the direction of a binge or purge. We have a strong support system in place and we are getting better at utilizing our supports rather than resorting to unhealthy behaviors. We continue to learn about ourselves and the disorder and we have an increasing capacity to cope with our feelings.

Ongoing Recovery is a process in which life is no longer dictated by crisis. We are more comfortable with food and our bodies, we are able to treat ourselves with love and respect, and we attract relationships where others have the capacity to do the same. We are able to set limits around people and situations which are unhealthy for us, and we can successfully cope with our emotions. We still rely on outside support for those times when we are overwhelmed by circumstances or emotion or when we feel the need to resort to unhealthy thinking or behaviors.

Carly: If I understand this correctly, it appears that each phase sort of builds off the other. Is it possible to be in between two phases at once?

Jillian: Absolutely! Remember recovery is not clear cut – that is why it can be so difficult.

Carly, I am pleased that you chose to discuss this concern here and we will continue to support each other along the way.

Is there anything else you would like to share?

Carly: No, not right now, thanks.

Jillian: Who would like to talk next about their week?

Anika: I've been thinking a lot about last week's discussion about feelings, and I decided writing them down was a good idea.

It has been kind of a difficult week with my family because they keep involving my aunt in all of my business. My mother keeps calling her to tell her about what I've been eating and how my new clothes are getting tight. I guess what I never realized before was how little privacy I have and how mad that makes me. There's no escaping them.

Taylor: Couldn't you just tell them all to butt out of your business? That would make me so mad!

Anika: I never really get mad at my family because I think that would make them more disapproving of me, and I spend so much time trying to please them. They think I'm too sensitive as it is.

They're all I have.

Jillian: Anika, it sounds very difficult for you to express your feelings and needs to your family. It also must be hard to hear you are too sensitive just because you feel.

Anika: Very.

Jillian: Anika, at your age and stage of development, having separate feelings within such a close family network can be very challenging – it is in most families – but it seems the cultural influences at play make it even harder. It is important to consider, however, that in maintaining their same viewpoints, you may be denying yourself of what you are really feeling and needing. Getting in touch with what is really going on can be difficult and overwhelming, but it is a big step in getting healthier.

I am glad you felt comfortable enough to share your discoveries with the group. You were very honest when you said that getting angry is not an option for you with your family – you want to please them. Anger is a particularly difficult emotion for people with eating disorders, perhaps for people in general, and especially for women. Many of us have never really learned to express feelings of anger freely, and most of us don't feel entitled to this feeling. For most people, they have also grown up in settings where others have not really learned to deal with their anger in a constructive way.

Anika: This is helpful. I am going to try and keep writing down my feelings, but I just cannot handle anymore disapproval from my family.

Jillian: I understand, Anika. I am hopeful that your writing will help you find a voice that you can be comfortable with to begin experimenting with expressing yourself to others.

Anika: Thank you.

Jillian: You are welcome.
   Min and Stephanie, you are particularly quiet. Is there anything that you wanted to add?

   Min begins to speak while looking down at the floor.

Min: No not really, but I do have a thought.

Jillian: Excuse me one moment, Min, I cannot hear you very well. If you are able, would you please speak up a bit.

   Min looks up and begins making eye contact with Jillian.

Min: I'm sorry. Yes of course I will try.
   Well it's just listening to this conversation, I'm thinking about how I work so hard at trying to ensure that I'm never going to do anything that will make my family disappointed in me, especially my father.

Jillian: If I understand correctly for you, this discussion is also bringing up feelings about your role in your family.

Min: Yes, I guess since I was very young, I've never felt consistently loved or accepted by my family. It always seems if I do what others want or what I know would please them, then I feel accepted. I feel so bad saying all this because I have a wonderful family. I mean my dad sent me to America for school so I would have many opportunities.

Why do I feel this way?

Jillian: Min, this need for love and acceptance from your family is very real. Your question is important and I would love to explore it further. It brings up an important subject I feel is very central to understanding recovery. I would like to explain about how this self critical part may exist for all of you.

We began our journey of recovery with a discussion about feelings. For many young women, like yourselves, with eating disorders, the challenge of maintaining emotional equilibrium in the wake of overwhelming situations and events in your lives seems impossible and can lead you to unhealthy ways of coping. However, there is more involved here than just managing your feelings. When we stop to examine the process of feeling more carefully, we can see there is another component at play. **Your feelings develop in response to the ideas, opinions, and beliefs you have about yourselves, people, and the world you live in.**

It is my viewpoint, and that of many others who have studied and written on the subject, that women who have eating disorders tend to see themselves in an incessantly critical and harshly unforgiving light. They carry with them a belief of being not good enough – of being unworthy of happiness, reward, and success. This is not to say they do not want these things – they feel undeserving of them. I call this perception that you, Min, and others may hold of yourselves **the voice of the eating disorder**. If you are constantly barraged with internal messages telling yourself that you are not good enough – you are not meeting the mark in nearly all areas of your lives – it is nearly impossible to maintain emotional equilibrium. If you believe you are unworthy, then you will feel unworthy.

Min: I find this very insightful. I never thought of this critical part of myself as a Voice that is related to my eating disorder. Could you please explain some more about this?

Jillian: **One of the most talked about characteristics that is so central to the experience of having an eating disorder, and critical to its understanding, is the notion of there being an inner voice which drives unhealthy behaviors.** Many authors who have written about eating disorders describe this phenomenon as a division of self. They explain that when you are struggling with an eating disorder, you often experience the presence of an overly critical inner voice. There also exists inside of you the more reasonable and understanding voice, but the critical voice tends to be more pervasive and influential.

My experience with girls in recovery groups has been that when they are in the throes of their disorder, their lives become consumed by the negative and harsh voice. This voice wants nothing less than to push them to a point that is well beyond what is healthy or reasonable for them. Their self-worth becomes determined by how many calories they restrict, how much they burn when exercising, and how much weight they lose. How they feel about themselves becomes directly tied to how well they feel they meet the demands of the eating disorder voice.

Min: This is helpful.

Carly: I don't really ever hear two separate voices inside of me. It's more this dark feeling of gloom that comes over me, and sometimes I don't even know why. It's often like I have let someone down, I haven't worked hard enough, or I am not measuring up. I am left feeling too lazy, too stupid, too boring, too intense, too fat, or too self absorbed for thinking about it so much – like I feel right now admitting this!

Jillian: Carly, what a great description of this voice. It sounds as if you are very familiar with the presence of this overly critical self even though you may not always be aware of receiving distinct and well-articulated messages.

The critical voice of the eating disorder can make you feel as though you are always under scrutiny, always questioning whether you are working to your true potential. Many girls feel they are not pretty enough, smart enough, athletic enough, or considerate enough. I have learned that numerous girls, even when acutely ill and hospitalized, don't feel they are even sick enough to have earned the true label of being eating disordered. And the flip side is true as well: in recovery, they are often unable to credit themselves with being vigilant enough in their efforts to get better.

Carly: Kind of like how I was in the beginning of this evening's group.

Jillian: That is a great example.

Taylor: I'm just going to step in here and say something.
My therapist in the past used to tell me I was very hard on myself and I should try to practice saying nice things to myself. Sometimes I try not to listen to the negative talk, but it's so distracting. I try to give myself positive messages, but it's like watching the news with its constant ticker tape of negative talk running across my brain. Sometimes I feel like I am in the middle of a battlefield between those two selves. I hate it!
I also think that sometimes this negative talk feels comforting and safe. Isn't that crazy?

Jillian: Taylor, you bring up an important point.
The challenge of getting healthy can be overwhelming and tiring at times – as your eating disorder can be. The difference is that when you give in to the demands of the disorder, you end up reinforcing the hold it has on you. With each binge, purge, or restrictive cycle you give in to, the harder it is to withstand the next time. I think it's important to note that when you begin trying to fight back, the eating disorder voice may feel that much more powerful. It may feel as if it has tightened its hold on you. This is when it can feel comforting and safe to you because change can be scary. However, every time you resist the temptation to give in to these thoughts or behaviors, you are empowering your healthier self, your true self.

Stephanie: I think it is so hard to give something up when it is one of the only things that offers any comfort and relief.

When my life feels out of control, I feel so much better if I can remind myself that yesterday I stuck to the "rules" I laid out for myself around my eating or exercising. It is one of the things I first think about when I wake up in the morning, and if I followed them, I am less afraid to face the day. I know it's not healthy.

Jillian: I understand that this feeling of control can be very comforting, especially when your life may seem unpredictable. However, as much as it can give you a sense of comfort and relief, it also misleads you into believing this is what's best for you and this is what your true self wants. You have found a place of comfort (or so it seems) within your world. Recovery is about beginning to challenge or step out of that place of comfort.

Stephanie: That sounds so overwhelming to even think about.

Jillian: Understandably so.

Remember this is a process and the more tools you gain by talking with others and learning about yourself, the less intimidating stepping out of this "place of comfort" may be.

Anika: Where do you think the critical voice comes from?

Jillian: You have asked such a great question, but unfortunately it is difficult to give just one simple explanation.

Some psychologists believe we develop this internal criticism as a result of having overly critical parents or caregivers; we go on to internalize these negative perceptions of ourselves. Many hypothesize that this sense of never being good enough or of living with a feeling of constant shame results from a previous trauma that we experienced. Others argue that this perception may be strictly bio-chemical in nature; that our brains are not functioning the way they're supposed to due to a chemical imbalance. And lastly, there are many who feel strongly that eating disorders stem from societal influences, that they're the outcome of a culture which totally overemphasizes competition, individual success, and physical perfection. I believe that for each individual, the critical voice probably originates from some combination thereof, but in varying proportions.

Anika: So then why is it that girls like us with eating disorder issues are so affected by this critical voice when many others have experienced pain and disappointment in their lives?

Jillian: Another excellent question, Anika! Let me explain.

Although there is not one theory that seems to adequately explain why people with eating disorders perceive themselves as critically as they do, there is considerable consensus that the perceptions they hold – not just of themselves, but of the world around them – are very similar. Many professionals think that people with eating disorders see the world and themselves in it differently than other people and that these perceptions, however skewed or distorted, lead to unhealthy behaviors.

Anika: So you are saying that this critical part affects us because of a combination of many things and because we have developed these eating disorder habits and thoughts that actually "feed" (sorry for using this word) this critical voice.

Jillian: Very well said.

Carly takes the blanket off and hangs it over the back of her chair.

Carly: I think I know where you are going with all this. Are you talking about body distortion?

Jillian: Yes, Carly, body distortion is part of it, but it goes beyond just how one sees their body. It is how you view everything.

I wonder if you would explain to the rest of the group what you mean by body distortion?

Carly: Well, people with eating disorders look at themselves and see something different than what's really there. They see themselves much larger than they are.

Jillian: Yes, and it is often the feelings of inadequacy or overall unworthiness that skew their body image. These feelings distort perception the same way a fun house mirror would. What I am talking about is not just the distorted view they hold of their bodies, but of the world in general. I call this type of thinking **cognitive distortion**.

Min: I'm not sure I understand what you mean by cognitive distortion. That sounds like a technical term of sorts.

Jillian: Min, it does sound very psychological. Let me explain.

There are different kinds of distortions – or misperceptions, if you will – but one particularly common one in women with eating disorders is called **black and white thinking**.

I think some of you have probably heard about the concept of black and white thinking, or perhaps you've heard it referred to as "all or nothing thinking" – both of these terms basically mean the same. With this type of thinking, perceptions are polarized, and there is little opportunity to view actions in terms of balance or compromise. For instance: you are in either a good mood or bad mood because you set high standards for yourself and you have either met those standards or, in your eyes, you have failed. There is no room for negotiation or explanation, no possibility of compromise.

Min: Thank you, Jillian. That makes more sense to me now.

Jillian: It is wonderful that you asked for a deeper understanding. This is very important in our group process.

I would like to explain a little more to you all about this "all or nothing thinking".

This perception which can also be thought of as a script becomes an ingrained way of thinking. For example, if you decided you had to complete all of next week's assignments before you would allow yourself to go to your friend's party, it would be difficult for you to then decide to only complete a couple of them, take a break, go to the party, and then complete the rest of them tomorrow without feeling like you were letting someone down. And, of course, that someone would be you. This type of thinking, once it starts, tends to pick up speed and velocity as it goes along. The incomplete assignment becomes criteria for you to begin thinking you are lazy, you always take the easier road, or you'll never pass the grade. A high percentage of the time, this fault-finding thinking will target a specific area of vulnerability, which, for many people, has to do with body, weight, or image. Also true for many people: once it finds a target, it stays! And so you become entrenched in negativity towards yourself and, perhaps, directed at the rest of your world.

Stephanie: What you described sounds just like what always happens with me. I always feel like there's a right way and a wrong way, and once I'm on a track, I can't seem to switch. If I try to, I feel so guilty.

I'll give you an example: I always feel like I have to go home on the weekends, but if I do, I miss out on important things that go on at school, and it's harder to meet people. See, my sister is really sick, and she's waiting for heart surgery, and my mother hates leaving her to go and do anything for herself. If I go home, my mom can go out for a little while and take a break.

Anika: Does your mom stay with her all the time?

Stephanie: Pretty much right now. She's been able to work in the past when my sister was well enough to go to school, but that hasn't happened for awhile.

Jillian: Stephanie, it sounds like you and your family have a lot to contend with.

You have given us a great example about how this *cognitive distortion* can play out in real life. Thank you.

Taylor: Whew, that sounds really rough. I'm surprised you can deal with all that. You are a much stronger chic than I am.

Stephanie: It's not that I'm strong. I've just lived like this since my sister was born.

Jillian: I appreciate you sharing so much of yourself with us, Stephanie. Things do sound very difficult at home, and you must feel very conflicted about pursuing your own independence. It looks like some strong emotions are coming up for you around your family.

Stephanie: Yes, you are correct, there are. My therapist and I have been working on the goal of creating more individuality for me despite all the issues at home. Journaling is helping when different feelings come up for me.

Jillian: It is encouraging that you have discovered a coping skill that is helping you as you work through this process with your therapist.

Does anybody have questions about what we have discussed up to this point?

Taylor: About the whole black and white thinking thing, it sounds a lot like the eating disorder voice. Are they the same? And what the hell can you do to get rid of them?

Jillian: Great question, Taylor.

Yes, the eating disorder voice and black and white thinking are alike in that they are a part of you – a way you have learned to think about yourself and the world – but not a way that is the healthiest. One idea to begin altering this thinking is to start creating a new script, one with a supportive and compassionate voice. Once you have begun reworking the old negative one, you can begin practicing with a new one.

Taylor: I'm not following you.

Jillian: Let me explain.

Let's call the new script of a supportive and compassionate voice **positive self-talk**. Positive self-talk is just what it sounds like: talking to oneself in a positive tone, which may sound like an easy task, but not when you're new to the language.

Many therapists who work in the field of eating disorders have found it extremely helpful to teach their clients how to talk to themselves in this way. They have discovered that by helping them learn to self-talk in a kinder more gentle tone, it helps them to foster a more forgiving and compassionate attitude toward themselves. With this kinder and gentler attitude, it then becomes easier to let go of disordered eating and to embrace healthy behaviors.

I realize some of these coping skills are rather abstract and may be hard to grasp.

Taylor: You can say that again. I mean talking to yourself in a positive way when you're feeling disgusting feels so fake.

Jillian: Your right, Taylor, it does. At first, it may feel as though you are being falsely reassuring, like you're an imposter, because you are not used to thinking this way, and it will most likely feel unnatural and foolish. But after a while, it becomes possible to live this way authentically.

Some people find it's too difficult to talk to themselves in a positive voice, so they imagine what they would say to a friend who needed their reassurance. They also imagine they are talking to themselves as though they were a young child who really needed their support.

Min: Can you please quickly show us how you might do that?

Jillian: I will, but let's take this a step further and try practicing it?

But first, Taylor, did my explanation help?

Taylor: I guess. I'm just gonna listen to what you are going to say now.

Jillian: Okay, Taylor.

Here is how this works.

Essentially, you want to first acknowledge what your negative thought is and then try to replace it with the positive thought. Chances are you'll need to repeat this several times before it begins to sink in and impact your mood. Does anyone want to volunteer to try this out?

Stephanie: I will.

Jillian: Can you try to create out loud what your negative self-talk would sound like?

Stephanie: Let me try.

I only think of myself, and I'm so selfish. I should be more grateful for what I have. I'm never going to be successful in my life. How could I be? People don't really like me. I should be going home this weekend to help out with my sister…I would have nothing to lose by going, because who would want to hang out with such an oaf anyway?

Jillian: Stephanie, thank you for being so honest about your personal negative talk.

Now, what if you tried turning this into positive talk?

Stephanie: I'm not sure that I can do what you are asking – but let me try.

Listen to me and how I tear myself up into little pieces. No one is worthy of that kind of self-punishment. I really do deserve to be happy and to have friendships. I am a good person who is learning to become more comfortable with myself and others. This takes time. If I stay at school this weekend, I will have an opportunity to practice these skills. I may not master the art of socializing right away, but I will get better at it over time. There is nothing wrong with taking care of myself. I'm worth it!

Jillian: Stephanie, you did amazing! Nice job.

Is this pretty clear for all of you or would you like to practice some more?

Min: That was really helpful, but could we please try one more example?

Jillian: Sure. Is there a critical voice you'd like to practice with?

Min: I didn't mean me.

Jillian: That's okay, Min. You don't have to if you don't want.

Min: Actually, I will try.

I hope this is okay. I can't help being really annoyed with myself for messing up this opportunity in school. My family worked so hard to get me into a good school, and I went ahead and blew it by almost getting kicked out.

How do I say anything positive to myself about that?

Jillian: Does anybody have any ideas?

Stephanie: I think you should tell yourself it's a really big adjustment being away from home for the first time, and even harder being in a new culture. You are obviously having a harder time getting accustomed to it than you thought you would, and it's coming out in different ways. It's a good thing you're trying to do something about your eating before it got any worse – or before you did get kicked out. Take my word for it, the longer you struggle with an eating disorder, the harder it is to get better. You are working on finding healthier ways to cope.

Min looks directly at Stephanie.

Min: Thank you, Stephanie. That was really helpful. I have never thought of talking to myself like that. It feels nice yet very uncomfortable.

Jillian: That is a great observation. When negative self-talk is what you are accustomed to, hearing positive words instead can feel very strange.

I think this is a really good time to tell all of you about another strategy that will help to make the practice of positive self-talk a little easier to comprehend and accept.

In the book **Radical Acceptance**, Tara Brach, meditation leader and psychologist, talks about how modern-day society – with its over focus on competition and individualism – has created a culture now infested with shame. She explains it is not just women with eating disorders who feel this ever-present cloak of unworthiness but people in general. The solution, she suggests, is to adopt an attitude of radical acceptance. This means, embracing yourself with the heart of a Buddha. Within Buddhist culture, there is a belief everyone has Buddha nature.

This means, essentially, everyone is born with innate goodness. In fact, in her book, Brach tells a story about how, several years ago, when the Dalai Lama came to the United States and was asked by a group of teachers and psychologists to talk about the suffering of self-hatred, he responded with a look of confusion and asked: "What is self-hatred?"

So, to embrace an attitude of "radical acceptance" implies to live with two wings. One wing is a wing of seeing – that is, being totally present and aware of what is going on for you. The other wing is the wing of compassion: treating yourself with kindness and care no matter what you've thought, felt, or done. The Buddhists believe that in order to fly (or live) freely, it is necessary to have both wings.

When Stephanie, you showed Min how to utilize the skill of positive self-talk, you were illustrating how to use radical acceptance. The wing of seeing was for Min to see her situation at school as it was really happening – the eating disorder behaviors were causing problems. The wing of compassion was for her to treat herself in an understanding and forgiving way, despite what was going on.

This is a lot to absorb all at once, so don't worry if you don't get it all. These ideas will continue to resonate throughout our groups.

Are there any questions?

Carly: I have one more question, but it's not exactly related.

You know how you said people with eating disorders have a lot of the same perceptions? Well, how do we know it's not the unhealthy behaviors that are contributing to the distortions?

Jillian: Carly, that is another good insight. I think many of the unhealthy eating behaviors tend to reinforce the cognitive distortions.

Once your body begins responding to your behaviors by becoming unhealthier or undernourished – your body chemistry is altered and the mind is definitely affected. It actually slows down. There was a study done in 1945 known as the *Minnesota Starvation Experiment* which was a study designed to evaluate the physiological and psychological effects of severe and prolonged dietary restriction. For a detailed discussion of the findings, you can either look up this study online or there is a lengthy text about it entitled *The Biology of Human Starvation*. What is particularly relevant about the study is that, in addition to the dramatic physiological changes the participants underwent while severely restricting their food intake, they also experienced some of the following psychological symptoms: a preoccupation with food, severe emotional distress, depression, and social withdrawal. Moreover, they also reported a significant decline in concentration, comprehension, and judgment.

Anika: This study is about starvation. Do these effects occur for people who use food like I do?

Jillian: Yes, this study's focus is on starvation and how it affects the body, but my experience has been that these symptoms are all very common in people who are restricting and /or bingeing and purging, and it is often difficult to distinguish what has caused what. Many girls have reported to me that when they are heavily involved in their disorder, their world feels as though it diminishes in size, to the extent that it becomes difficult to think of anything besides food, weight, and numbers.

Does this clarify your question, Anika?

Anika: Yes, thank you.

Jillian: We have discussed a lot here this evening. So I would like to take this time to discuss some more coping skills that may help with some of the internal struggles each of you may be dealing with.

I would like to begin by talking about **affirmations**. Affirmations are positive, self-affirming phrases. Numerous women with eating disorders have found that in conjunction with using positive self-talk to counter the eating disorder voice, it is very helpful to have these self-affirming phrases on hand to repeat to themselves. When someone is in emotional distress, it can be difficult to come up with one's own words of reassurance at that time. Therefore, it's helpful to have comforting words on hand – either some you have composed ahead of time or others written by someone else.

The words you choose to use should be capable of countering the false beliefs or unrealistic expectations you hold for yourself at that specific point in time. Some people actually write their affirmations down on index cards and take them along when they think they will be in a situation that could be particularly stressful. Others will carry a stone or wear a piece of jewelry which to them symbolizes their affirming thought – almost as a reminder or a life jacket, if you will.

I have developed a list of some examples of affirmations, but you might want to write or create your own to be able to tailor them to your individual needs. Relax for a moment as I read these to you. Please close your eyes if you wish and sit comfortably.

I am just fine as I am, and I don't need to be perfect

I am strong and capable

I deserve to take the time and space to be healthy

I am entitled to my feelings – good or bad, angry or sad

I have accomplished many important things in my life

With the help and support of those I trust, I can get through this

I have the necessary tools to cope with this

I can discover what I'd like to change about myself without losing sight of my self-worth

If I don't do everything as I had originally planned, I'm no less a person and no less desirable

I am capable of achieving what I want in my life

I am safe

There will be people in my life that think I'm great and others who won't

I am resilient

I don't have to measure my beauty in terms of cultural standards

Min: Jillian, thank you for reading those phrases. They are really
nice.

I hope I can begin to believe these types of phrases.

Jillian: Just the fact that you are expressing appreciation for the
kindness these words project is a positive step for you.

Remember, this is your process.

Min: I will try.

Jillian: I would like to now talk to you all about one more coping
skill this evening. This is my personal favorite because I believe
it creates space for us to grow, think, and exist. In other words
it can create options. This is the concept of **rainbow thinking**.
The idea originated from ***The Don't Diet, Live-It Workbook*** as
a strategy to help counter black and white thinking. If we look
at black and white thinking as polarized and inflexible, then
rainbow thinking is a middle of the road way of seeing things.
It provides us with a lens with which to view the world and
ourselves in an array of colors. By doing this, we are positioned
better and are more apt to set reasonable expectations for
ourselves and others. When what life dishes out to us appears
to be more reasonable and palatable, we are less apt to feel the
pull to resort to unhealthy coping mechanisms. I have two
vignettes for all of you which will help illustrate the usage of
rainbow thinking.

Let's take a moment and I will read them.

Vignette One

It's recess on a typical school day. Jenn is with a
group of her friends in the hallway, having an intense
conversation about another friend, Amy, who is not
there. Jenn has been concerned about Amy lately because she hasn't been acting like herself. She has been

short-tempered and irritable. Jenn feels these friends are being unfair and insensitive to Amy, and she makes a comment in Amy's defense. In response to Jenn's comment, Eric and Joe criticize her for being a drama queen. Jenn returns to class feeling hurt and humiliated. She is unable to concentrate and begins feeling really horrible about herself. Negative and self-doubting thoughts fill her head: "I'm stupid. My friends don't like me, they only tolerate me. Maybe I do say things just for a reaction. I hate the way I look today. If I wasn't so damn plain looking, no one would jump down my throat because I dare to offer my opinion."

Jenn became quickly caught up in a downward spiral of black and white thinking. She immediately jumped to the conclusion that she was not liked and unworthy of friendship. She saw herself in the wrong and her peers as right.

If she had been utilizing the skill of rainbow thinking, she would have been able to see this one comment didn't necessarily characterize the nature of the entire friendship. Perhaps Eric and Joe were being totally insensitive – which they could be at times – but they were basically good guys. Maybe she did see situations with people in a more sensitive and empathic way, but this doesn't make her unlikable or unworthy. In fact, maybe it makes her more special.

Now I will read the second one.

Vignette Two

I woke up for school the other morning and I was determined that the day was going to be a perfect day, the start of a new beginning. I showered and went downstairs for breakfast. I had decided that I was going to try to eat a small but sensible breakfast, because that's what I was supposed to do. I ate my planned meal and then, without even really thinking, took some more yogurt. I began to feel awful. I felt guilty, and I felt like I was a failure. I actually heard the words in my head: "You will be fat forever." I wanted to crawl back into bed and forget the morning ever happened. But I really couldn't afford to miss another day of school. I decided to get dressed, but everything I put on looked awful. I imagined the extra helping of yogurt made me look bigger.

This was going nowhere fast, and I couldn't stand it anymore. I shouted "STOP!" to myself several times over and over. I didn't really eat that much for breakfast. And besides, if I want to recover, I have to keep challenging myself. I'm not a bad person. I deserve to eat and be nurtured. It's part of being human. I need to sustain myself. I have a very busy day ahead of me. All right, so I had two extra tablespoons of yogurt. It's not that big a deal. I don't always have to be perfect. This I can take control of and continue to work on. I can decide how I choose to cope with these challenges. I finished getting ready and left for school.

Anika: Rainbow thinking seems very liberating. I really enjoyed these examples – thank you.

Jillian: I'm glad you enjoyed them.

My hope is that with all the information I will be giving you during our groups, each of you will find bits and pieces that suit you best and help you as you continue on your journey of recovery. Just by being here every week, each of you is getting a "travel bag" for this journey full of new skills that you can use whenever you need.

Before we end this week's group, I would like to discuss one more thing. I would like to present each of you with the idea of a *Weekly Self Challenge*. In previous groups, the girls have found it particularly helpful to use the time in between our sessions to practice changing the way they would typically do things, to consider our discussion from the week before and commit to challenging themselves by trying out healthier thinking or behaviors. They had discovered that by utilizing the safety and structure of the group format, they were less fearful and more motivated to make changes they had been unable to make before. They had also found it helpful, prior to closing the group for that current week, to consider out loud what they would each commit to.

So, in considering this week's discussion and attempting to continue to encourage you all, I would like to encourage you, this week only, to challenge yourself by experimenting with some of the new ideas we have discussed this evening. This can be done by using last week's Daily Check-In list to assist your journaling process, practicing positive self talk, utilizing affirmations, or simply by creating your own challenge. When we come together next week, for our third week, we will have the opportunity to discuss your challenge and how it went if you wish. The idea is if you find this experience of challenging yourself between our time together each week is helpful, please continue to do this for the following weeks we will be meeting.

Does anyone have any ideas about what they would like their weekly self-challenge to be?

Min: I do. I think I'd like to try talking to myself more positively and maybe try not to purge.

Carly: For me, I'm going to try to be easier on myself. I have a lot of school work this week.

Jillian: Thank you both for sharing your challenges.
Does anybody else feel comfortable enough to share?

Taylor: To be honest with you, I'm not really sure what to do. Could I just think about it and get back to you next week?

Jillian: Sure, Taylor.
Remember, please use our group how it feels best for each of you. This may fluctuate from week to week. This experience

in our group is and will continue to be individual for all of you.
Stephanie and Anika, would either of you like to share with the group your challenge?

Stephanie: I guess I'll write in my journal more and I would like to practice rainbow thinking.

Anika: Writing sounds like a good idea. I also think I will be thinking about those vignettes more over the week.

Jillian: I wish you all the best as each of you carry out your self-challenges during this week. I want to thank you for your honesty and courage during our group. It has been a pleasure being here with all of you this evening. I would now like to read the *Words of Hope*. Sit back and relax, close your eyes if you wish as you absorb this inspirational thought.

I want each of you to know I think recovery from an eating disorder is possible. Being able to acknowledge the presence of your internal dialogue and discovering its pattern is a powerful defense against it. Your ongoing challenge will be in learning how to strengthen your healthier voice and belief in your own worthiness, but this is entirely possible. There will be a time when the affirmations that you recite faintly and in disbelief will become part of a chorus of celebratory song that lives inside of you.

Have a wonderful week.

Perfectionism

Perfectionism is an issue that is a very common struggle for those who have an eating disorder. **Young women who wrestle with Anorexia, Bulimia, or Binge-eating disorder experience the world as being made up of *shoulds, musts, ought to*s, and *have to*s living by a rigid set of rules.**

Many times, these girls are driven by external pressures which can include acting a certain way and chasing after insurmountable standards. There is also the cultural expectation of body flawlessness. With all of this combined, it often results in these young women feeling they are never good enough or attractive enough.

Within my experience, I have found anxiety is at the core generating these thoughts of not being good enough. The struggle of perfectionism is reinforced by the voice of the eating disorder. Often these girls believe that their eating disorder can make them perfect, and if they are perfect they will be loved, accepted, and happy. They strive to become the most attractive, best student, most popular, most seductive, and best daughter. For many girls, their worth is based on these pressures of being enough, doing enough, and looking good enough. This over the top drive for perfectionism oftentimes reinforces eating disorder behaviors and can make recovery more challenging.

Managing Perfectionism

For many young women struggling with an eating disorder, learning to nurture themselves through **relaxation and meditation can be helpful in their recovery process.** As they slow down and look inward, they are often able to listen and see what they may really need and want. I encourage them to begin nurturing themselves in a kind, compassionate way.

For many young women, using these self care tools appears to turn the volume down on some of the pressures they are enduring. This then allows them to no longer base their thoughts and actions on what the external world wants and expects of them. It becomes possible to now allow themselves to do what they can, as best they can, for the type of day or moment they may be having.

Have you ever noticed how many times in one day you feel like you are not being enough, doing enough, or looking good enough? Do you have an idea where your desire for perfection stems from? What does it mean for you? What can it offer you? As you work through your own journey of recovery you can begin to notice the "perfect in the imperfect". This can be very liberating and often occurs as you learn new, healthier ways to nurture and acknowledge yourself without all of your own personal *shoulds*, *musts*, *ought to*s, and *have to*s.

> I have spent my whole life feeling as though I have to be perfect at everything I do. I get so sick of it, but if I don't give something one hundred percent, I feel like I'm slacking.
>
> **–Carly**

Jillian: Welcome back. This is the third week of our group. I want all of you to know I really enjoy spending this time with you every week. I feel a strong, positive energy in this room when we come together. I see this as a true reflection of all of you.

Let's spend some time checking in on how everyone is doing. I have been wondering how each of you fared experiencing your challenges. What was the week like for you?

Min: If it's okay, I can start.

Taylor: Min, I don't mean to interrupt – I know it's rude, but your hair looks awesome. What did you have done to it?

Min: Thank you, Taylor. I tried getting it layered to help deal with it being so thick.

Taylor: It looks awesome! Maybe I will try that with my hair – but mine isn't nice and thick like yours. It actually falls out at times. According to my wonderful doctor this happens because of my eating disorder – whatever. Anyway, sorry for the interruption.

Min: That's okay. I appreciate your compliment. I have been very nervous about this change. I have kept my hair the same for many years.

Enough about my hair. I would like to tell you all about my week. I have had a really good week. My sister has been here from New York, where she goes to school, and we've done a lot of talking. I don't get a chance to see her that often, and we never really talked before about the whole eating thing. She gave me a lot of advice about how to eat more healthfully and about portions, and she told me if I eat reasonably and exercise moderately, I won't have to worry. So, I'm trying it, and so far it seems to be working. In fact, I haven't even purged after any meals.

Jillian: That is wonderful, Min, that seeing your sister was such a positive experience for you. It appears visiting with your sister may have helped you be able to carry out your challenge for yourself by receiving her support.

Min: Yes, she definitely did.
That's really all for now.

Jillian: Okay, who wants to share next?

Carly: That's really great, Min!
For me, things aren't going that well. Because I haven't been able to exercise with my team, I'm feeling a lot like a fat slug. My challenge for the week was to try using some positive self-talk by telling myself the reason I was feeling this way was because I have a tendency to exaggerate any changes I feel in my body. My individual therapist even says I imagine myself getting bigger after I eat something I feel guilty about or when I feel guilty for not working out. So, I guess I've been having a hard time with all these feelings. I imagine everyone around me can see my body changing, and then I obsess about what to wear or try to hide it, and half the time I don't even want to go out for fear someone will see me. And then I feel like I want to scream and cry, and I have trouble catching my breath. I hate all this and I'm so sick of feeling this way! Oh, and also there is this boy I've been seeing, and he just doesn't get it. He thinks I'm totally crazy for worrying about my weight – but then I have to listen to him and his friends talk about all the "hotties" there are on campus! Maybe the reason I'm so emotional right now is because I'm getting my period.

Stephanie: So much of what you just described sounds like what goes on inside of me. It's amazing how you can talk about it so openly. People around you just don't get it. They think you can just stop worrying at will. They don't realize that once there's something that just doesn't feel right, it's hard to think of anything else.

Does your boyfriend know you have an eating disorder?

Jillian: Stephanie, sorry to interrupt, but please hold onto your question for Carly for one moment.

I just want to back up and make a couple of comments about some things you said, Carly and Stephanie.

Have you and your therapists ever discussed the fact that oftentimes anxiety and obsessive thinking can go hand in hand with an eating disorder?

Stephanie: Yes, we have discussed how so much of my anxiety about life and its out of control circumstances definitely has an effect on my eating disorder.

Jillian: Well said. I am glad, Stephanie, that you have explored this.

I asked you girls this because many people believe strongly that anxiety is at the root of an eating disorder or that is can exist alongside of it. When you begin to examine some of the underlying issues behind an eating disorder, you realize there is a lot more to them than just food and weight.

During our groups I am certain we will continue uncovering some of the attitudes and perceptions that contribute to eating issues, and then ultimately examine additional ways to promote healing.

Carly, how about you, have you every discussed anxiety with your therapist?

Carly: Yeah, I have been told in the past that they think I have Obsessive-Compulsive Disorder and panic attacks, but I've been scared to take any medication. And I guess part of me believes I can actually overcome this myself if I work hard enough.

Stephanie, to answer your question, no my boyfriend doesn't know yet. I don't want to scare him off. We've only been dating a short time.

Anika: Sorry to interrupt but I would just like to ask if I may, what is Obsessive-Compulsive Disorder, and what is the connection between anxiety and eating disorders?

Jillian: Great question, Anika. As I answer your question, I think it will help further explain some of what Carly was saying.

Obsessive-Compulsive Disorder, OCD, is a disorder many people believe is caused by a chemical imbalance in the brain. When researchers have studied this disorder by taking images of the brain, they have actually been able to demonstrate how the brain of someone with OCD looks different from someone who doesn't have it. This structural difference does not cause medical concern. However, it usually causes a person to experience repetitive thoughts or behaviors they feel unable to control. Many of these repetitive thoughts are connected to things or situations they worry about. They then feel a need to engage in repetitive acts to help them alleviate the anxiety. For example, one of the most well known compulsions is repetitive hand washing. This compulsion usually occurs because a person has overwhelming anxiety related to germs and illness. The act of washing their hands is a way they have adapted to control their obsessive worry about germs. By washing their hands, they feel they have gained some control over their fear of becoming ill.

People can have these obsessive worries about many different things. This relates to Anorexia, Bulimia, and Binge-eating disorder because many people feel strongly that it is a person's underlying anxiety actually fueling their repetitive concern with food, weight, and body image. The obsessive concern then fuels the behaviors.

Anika: So anxiety acts like a spark to start and keep the eating disorder going?

Jillian: It could, for instance, if you have an underlying fear of gaining weight, you are more likely to engage in repetitive behaviors you believe will reduce the chances of your gaining weight. In fact, in Aimee Liu's recent book, *Gaining*, she discusses this correlation between OCD and eating disorders and states the following statistic: two-thirds of the people diagnosed with Anorexia and one-third of those diagnosed with Bulimia have OCD. This finding strongly suggests there is a physiological component to the disorder and highlights the fact anxiety plays an important role here. What's more, it suggests, the imbalance of chemicals in the brain are causing these worries and behaviors, making it that much harder to just will them away.

Anika: I've never realized how powerful feeling anxious can be!

Carly: Definitely. All these obsessive thoughts and the nervousness that goes with them suck, but my therapist and I work on this almost every week.

Jillian: I am glad you and your therapist do work on this topic because along with being overwhelming, it can be exhausting to deal with this every day.

Carly: Yes it is!

Jillian: How about you, Stephanie, is there anything you wanted to share about your week?

Stephanie: Well, it's been a pretty difficult week because I have some big papers due and everyone in my class is so stressed. I'm really tired because I've been up late doing research, and I haven't been doing that well with my meals. My challenge for the week was to try to talk to myself and remind myself not to get too worked up about exams, but it hasn't been working. I guess it's like one of those obsessions you talked about. I get really anxious about not doing well on tests, and so I never feel like I've studied enough.

Jillian: It sounds as though you've been under a lot of pressure, not only pressure related to school but pressure coming from the added responsibility of having to report to the group about your meals and weekly challenge. I'm glad you were able to share this.

Were you able to write in your journal?

Stephanie: A little, but it takes time and I felt so guilty writing in a journal when I have these huge research papers to complete.

Jillian: I understand, it sounds very busy for you right now. Just do what you can in those moments – even if you only take five minutes to journal, it may help you stay connected to yourself when your life is so demanding.

Stephanie: Thanks, just hearing you say that makes it seem a bit more doable.

Jillian: I'm glad, Stephanie.

How about you, Taylor, how was your week?

Taylor: Well, to tell you the truth, I forgot about the weekly challenge thing, but I've had a pretty good week. This is shocking! My boyfriend and I got back together, so this seems to be putting me in a much better mood.

Jillian: Taylor, at the last group you hadn't decided on a challenge for yourself, so you didn't forget to do it.

Taylor: That's right. Thanks for reminding me. I was wondering why I couldn't remember what I said I would do.

Jillian: It is important that you are able to acknowledge that your week went well and you are feeling better.

Taylor: Thanks.

Jillian: Anika, how about your week?

Anika: I've had a pretty good week. I was offered a paid internship for the Summer, which I'm really happy about, and I've been writing a lot in a journal and thinking a lot about my feelings. I'm noticing I tend to want to binge when I want or need something I don't have. So instead of bingeing, I'm using writing to help me figure out what I'm wanting.

Jillian: That's really great, Anika. You have made an important discovery for yourself that also holds true for many people with eating disorders: If you look carefully behind the behaviors, there are usually feelings and needs being overlooked.

Was there anything in particular you found you were feeling?

Anika: A lot of anger toward my parents for criticizing and judging me so much. And I guess lately I've been kind of lonely. I thought my loneliness resulted from my wanting to be in a relationship, but I realized I would also like the companionship of other girls my age.

Jillian: Those are very insightful discoveries about yourself. It is important to praise yourself for choosing to begin learning more about who you are and what you need, although, this may not always be easy.

When we make room in our lives to pay attention to how we're really feeling, unfortunately, we can also uncover some painful needs and emotions. However, if you address them with care, it is these very revelations that will help you recover.

I'm sorry things at home have been so tough for you, Anika.

Anika: I appreciate your caring. For the first time in a long time, when I come here I feel like I can be myself and I will be respected.

Jillian: I hope this group offers every one of you the opportunity to discover and /or meet some of your needs that have been pushed aside for a long time.

I wonder if any of you have ever studied Abraham Maslow's *Hierarchy of Needs*? This is a famous study that was done back in 1943 on human development. It is frequently referred to because it uncovered the important fact that, as human beings, in order for us to be able to grow and flourish, we have certain basic needs which have to be met. These include: the need to be fed, to be sheltered and safe, to be loved and supported, and the need for friendship. He went on to explain that for humans to develop and expand intellectually and emotionally, it is essential to have these fundamental needs in place.

Many of us may see these needs as merely self-indulgent desires, or we have been told by others they are as such, so we tend to ignore them or minimize their importance. Many people with eating disorders are unaccustomed to having needs. They have feared them and defended against them so vigilantly that they are no longer attuned to their presence. However, needs are part of who we are, and as we slowly learn to uncover and address them, we can continue to grow to meet our fullest potential.

Because it is so common for women with eating disorders to become disconnected from their needs, which prevents them from then being able to recognize them, I have developed a list that has been helpful for many girls in my previous groups. When you're upset or feeling pulled to use behaviors, it might be helpful for you to think of this list and explore what could be missing.

I will read this list to you and when I am done, I welcome any questions or comments any of you may have. Please try and allow yourselves to relax as I read this list and allow the words and their meanings to permeate you.

Some Examples of What You Might Need
To be loved
To be heard
To be active
To feel safe
To laugh

To be silly

To be encouraged

To cry

To create

To be challenged

To do nothing

To walk on the beach

To pray

To be forgiven

To be angry

To be held

To scream

Min: That is a really great list.

I do have one question if that is okay.

Jillian: What is your question?

Min: Why do you think we are so fearful of having needs?

Jillian: I think this is a very helpful question when you all are here attempting to discover healthier thoughts and behaviors for yourselves.

A lot of it has to do with those overwhelming feelings we talked about earlier. When connecting with them in the first place led you to feeling as though you were drowning, you learned it wasn't safe to feel them. For others, perhaps, as I indicated before, you have been taught at some time that your needs came with too high a price – you may have been berated or judged for having them.

Anika: So, basically we are afraid of our needs and what goes along with them.

Jillian: Yes, Anika, well said.

Min, does this answer your question?

Min: It does. I'm going to keep thinking about this some more.

Jillian: It is important that this is something you are willing to begin exploring.

All of this conversation has brought up some thoughts in me I would like to share with all of you that I hope will be helpful.

Over the past couple of weeks, we've been talking a lot about the voice of the eating disorder – how when you have an eating disorder you tend to view the world in very polarized ways and how this perception then creates a set of expectations that you may place on yourself. Essentially, these expectations that you hold for yourself are rules – stringent standards you may feel you must meet in order for yourself to feel you are of value. There is nothing wrong with having goals to live by or with having codes or moral ethics – they help keep you safe and on track. However, when your sole mission in life becomes a never-ending quest to see how close you can come to **perfection**, you may be blind-sided into believing this is a priority for your happiness and success. The very fabric of your day can become an infinite ream of reminder notes and to-do lists. You are constantly judging yourself to determine whether the things you've said and done are flawless enough. You may review, incessantly, what you have overlooked or left out of place.

A lot of people consider themselves to be perfectionists, and they battle the mental, physical, and spiritual exhaustion which can go along with this trait, but for people with eating disorders, the standard for perfection comes with an even higher price. Their high standards prevail in all areas of functioning – social, emotional, and intellectual – but reigns most heavily in the food, weight, and body image arenas. As a result of this standard, women with eating disorders are forced to trade in health and happiness for their never-ending pursuit of flawlessness.

Carly: I can really relate to what you are saying and it is really hard.

Jillian: It is. In fact, let's all take a moment to pause from our discussion. This is a lot to think about. I would like to share this excerpt with all of you from same book I mentioned earlier this evening. In her book *Gaining*, Liu writes of her peers with eating disorders:

> My fellow dieters and I had always been compliant, helpful, studious, and orderly; and except for our stubborn refusal to eat, we retained those qualities. Even at our thinnest, we excelled in our studies. Many of us were talented artists, writers, musicians, or dancers. Our teacher praised us and our parents boasted about us even as they lamented or rebuked us for our obstinacy.

I would like to just sit and let what I just read settle.

The room becomes so quiet that the clock ticking on the book shelf can be heard.

Taylor: This silence sucks, I'm sorry; I cannot stand when nobody is talking, and how that clock sounds. Its ticking is so annoying!

Jillian: I can put it away, Taylor, if you find it distracting.

Taylor: I just can't stand the noise.

Jillian: I respect that you were able to let me know what you needed in this moment of silence.

Taylor: Thanks, even though it feels a little strange to hear you say that.

Jillian: If everyone is done digesting this, I have a question. I'm wondering, as we go around the room for the check-in as we begin each week, whether or not you are able to hear in each other the exceedingly high expectations you place on yourselves?

I would like all of you at this time to stop and consider what the unspoken rules you hold for yourselves are? What are the *should*s, *must*s, *ought to*s and *have to*s you must satisfy for you to feel complete?

I know this may feel overwhelming, but is there anyone who feels comfortable enough to share what they think their list of rules might look like? Feel free to take a minute to think about them or even write them down.

Stephanie: I'll take a stab at it.

I must get A's and be a good student. I have to be a good roommate and avoid conflicts. I have to be there for my friends when they need me. I shouldn't be too vain or only think of myself. I should be a good daughter. I have to eat and exercise as planned. I have to make something great of my life. I have to be politically correct. Around boys, I can't be too smart or assertive or they'll be intimidated. But I also can't be too ditsy.

I guess I'll have to think about the rest.

Jillian: Well done, Stephanie. I wonder what that was like for you?

Stephanie: I feel like now I shouldn't have so many shoulds.

I guess it makes me kind of sad that I do this to myself and that so many girls end up getting so sick because of the pressure they put on themselves.

Jillian: Your thoughts are very real and compassionate. Thank you for offering all that you just did to the group with your personal list of shoulds and your thoughts.

Stephanie: I think it's kind of funny because I am finding the talking we do here is helping me figure out parts of myself I never really understood.

Jillian: That's wonderful, Stephanie.

Carly: For me, this idea of perfection plagues me constantly.

What I mean is I have spent my whole life feeling as though I have to be perfect at everything I do. I get so damn sick of it, but if I don't give something one hundred percent, I feel like I'm slacking. Even when I do give something my all, I feel like I could have done better. When the eating disorder voice really gets going, I want to be the best anorexic ever! I drive myself and the people around me crazy.

Jillian: I can understand what you are saying. It seems like the idea of being perfect is a big struggle for you.

I know this may not be too comforting, but I think most of us in this room and many young women can relate to what you have just expressed. After all, we live in a culture preoccupied with outcomes. Don't misunderstand – results are important, but we spend a lot more time being concerned with the final product than with the actual process. In other words, we exercise not so much because we enjoy it, but for the end result. The same holds true for dieting. We diet thinking it will be a quick fix, not because we want to live a healthier lifestyle. We emphasize the importance of grades rather than making the act of learning the higher priority. We believe the deceptive message: One has to be the best at something in order to achieve recognition or success in life. This creates a climate of comparison, competition, and pressure to be the prettiest, make the most money, have the best grades, etc. When it comes to our bodies, we create stringent rules which are impossible for us to meet, without our becoming physically ill.

Taylor: Don't forget emotionally ill, too!

Jillian: Great point, Taylor!

Stephanie: Do you have any other suggestions for how to create kinder, gentler, and more reasonable expectations?

Jillian: I do.

One of the best ways to create kinder, gentler, more reasonable expectations is through offering ourselves self-nurturance. More and more, women, who for so many centuries have been the primary caregivers or nurturers of the home and family, are now part of the workforce or pursuing careers without the support of extended family or community. True, men have taken over a lot of the responsibilities of child-rearing and housekeeping, and for them, I'm certain this comes with its own set of challenges. But for women, providing care is an innate sense – one that is difficult to fully delegate or hand off to another person. As women, we remain vigilantly attentive to others even when they are not physically in our presence. In addition, women are caring more and more for aging parents.

Anika: Being a woman is very overwhelming!

Jillian: I agree Anika.

With all of this added responsibility, women are finding they are more exhausted and stressed out than ever before. The list of *should*s and *ought to*s has grown even longer. I am talking about this here because, as women, when we spend most of our time and energy trying to accommodate all of the needs of others, we begin to lose sight of what we really need and want. When we spend vast amounts of time trying to figure out what everyone around us needs, we lose us in the process. I believe an important part of recovery from an eating disorder involves learning to reconnect with your own true set of needs and desires – giving care to yourselves.

Now that I have elaborated about this kinder way of relating to ourselves I wonder, what comes to mind for any of you when we talk about self-care or self-nurturance?

Stephanie: For me I think of paying attention more to my own voice and what I need instead of everyone else.

Jillian: Stephanie, you have really hit the nail on the head! Yes, this is learning to nurture oneself. If you don't stop to listen, it is difficult to know what you need. Think for a moment about the dictionary definitions of nurturance:
  1. *To feed or nourish.*
  2. *To raise or promote the development of.*
  3. *All the environmental factors, collectively, to which the individual is subjected from conception onward.*
Self-nurturance is like learning to parent yourself in a compassionate and attentive way. Many of us don't really know

what this involves, and we have to learn as we go along. We must discover how to pay attention to our emotional needs, our physical needs, our intellectual needs, and our spiritual needs.

Let me explain a little further. In other words, caring for your physical self means evaluating whether you are getting enough rest, checking in with yourself to determine whether you have been sick long enough to warrant a visit to the doctor, assessing how hungry you are, looking at what you are eating to determine if you have a balanced diet, etc.

Your emotional needs have to do with your feelings: Are you being neglected? Are you sad, angry, or perhaps frightened? Are there ample opportunities in your day to check in with yourself to find out how you're really doing, or are there enough outlets for self-expression?

Your intellectual needs have to do with whether or not you are feeling mentally stimulated or challenged. Going to the movies, reading, or visiting museums are some ways of satisfying this.

Our spiritual needs are a little more difficult to describe, and they are very individual. For some people, spirituality pertains to religion, and for others, this realm can be satisfied through their relationships with people or with nature.

Min: I don't mean to interrupt, but do all these needs occur independently of each other?

Jillian: No Min, they do not, and thank you for making that point.

I don't mean to imply that these different areas are all separate. In fact, they are very much interrelated. What you do intellectually can also affect you spiritually and vice versa. By tending to these different parts of yourself, you are nurturing yourself – something we all need in order to be healthy.

I have a creative idea. Why don't we all brainstorm and put together a list of self-nurturing activities that may fulfill some of these needs I just spoke of. We will take turns by going around our circle. Carly, we will begin with you.

Carly: Listening to music, singing, dancing, and writing music.

Taylor: My turn, great.

I was wondering, can buying new shampoos and makeup and trying them out be one.

Jillian: Absolutely!

Keep going.

Taylor: I also want to add getting a manicure and massage.

Min: These are some things I like to do. I hope they are what you are asking me for – going for a long walk, doing a craft project, visiting friends, and visiting a book store.

Jillian: Well done, Min.

Anika, it's your turn.

Anika: Scrapbooking, taking a drive to a pretty place, taking a dog on a walk.

Stephanie: I've done some of this with my therapist.

Some of the self-nurturing activities I enjoy are writing in a journal, taking a hot bath, and even sometimes watching television (but not shows that make me feel bad about myself – I try to stay away from that).

Jillian: Thank you all. What productive work you all did.

These are all beautiful ways to care for yourselves. I hope you all can keep some of these nurturing ideas with you and maybe even try them out.

Now that we have completed this list, I would like to talk with all of you about **balance**.

It is my belief that in order for a person to be happy, healthy, and feel fulfilled, life needs to contain a certain amount of balance. This means that once we have an inkling of what our emotional, intellectual, physical, and spiritual needs are, we create opportunities to satisfy these needs. Unfortunately, however, because we spend so many of our waking hours tending to the needs of others, we are usually the last ones to recognize what we need or to recognize when we are off-kilter in some way.

So many women go through their lives functioning as well as they can (as extraordinary students, friends, athletes, employees, wives, mothers, etc.) while living within an imbalanced state. If we continue to function within this state of disequilibrium long enough, most of us will usually reach a point where we are forced to pay attention to our needs. Either we become physically and emotionally exhausted, or we develop physical complaints such as, headaches, backaches, stomachaches, problems sleeping, etc. Many of us become depressed, and often times we resort to using drugs, alcohol, or food so we can cope with our lives.

Stephanie: Why is it when you struggle with an eating disorder, does this balance you talk about seem so unattainable.

Jillian: I am glad you have noticed this, Stephanie. Let me explain.

It seems women with eating disorders are particularly prone to living in a state of imbalance because they tend to be the caregivers, they are often perfectionitstic, and, as we have previously discussed, it is not uncommon for them to be detached from the thoughts and feelings which might signal a problem.

Anika: So what you're saying is having such high self standards, and always trying to please others gets in the way of noticing what is going on within ourselves.

Jillian: Yes. Let us examine, for a moment, how perfectionism relates to imbalance.

When our motivation is to achieve perfection in one area of our lives, it usually requires our taking time and energy away for another area. At times, this is necessary. There are times when life situations demand this, like when someone we care about is extremely ill or we are trying to meet a deadline for work. However, it's important to realize that if we are continually placing this expectation on ourselves to be the perfect student, athlete, daughter, etc., we leave little time and energy for that worthwhile person inside. We create deficits in these other important areas.

Anika: That makes a lot to sense to me.

Jillian: I want you all to realize the challenge in recovery is to seek out balance in your life – but without making yourself crazy about it. This means at times gently letting go of things that cannot be attended to. There is a wonderful book by Alice Domar, Ph.D and Henry Dreher (*Self Nurture: Learning to Care for Yourself as Effectively as You Care for Everyone Else*) about learning to self-nurture. In it, they quote leading mind-body specialist Joan Borysenko by saying: "The only time you reach a perfect state of balance is when you are dead." I don't mean this to seem morbid. But in other words, we need to develop reasonable expectations about being balanced. Domar also explains that this is why it is important not to base self-nurturing on external rules and fantasies – the *should*s and *must*s. She advises her patients: "Proceed with certain qualities of mind and heart: awareness rather than impulsiveness; gentleness rather than militance; flexibility rather than rigidity; desire rather than obligation."

Min: I really like this quote. It seems so self forgiving to me.

Jillian: Very well said.

Another great source, I have already brought up from time to time, is *The Don't Diet, Live-It Workbook* and I would like to share it with you again because it discusses creating balance in our lives. LoBue and Marcus talk about adapting a **Live-It** as a way of life, to help to promote balance. They feel strongly that diets don't work for people because they are thought of as temporary and lead people to feel frustrated, preoccupied, and deprived. A Live-It, on the other hand, is about caring for yourself: eating a balanced diet, getting a moderate amount of exercise to be healthy, and attending to your mental, emotional, and spiritual needs. The authors equate these different spheres with the legs of a chair and go on to explain that when one leg is broken, the chair becomes imbalanced and unable to stand. They explain that it is much easier to maintain a strong, balanced chair-of- life if all needs are adequately being acknowledged. It is no accident that when we are feeling emotionally injured or physically depleted, we often resort to chocolate, restricting, or purging as a way to compensate for the imbalance.

Taylor: Now, this example makes more sense for me, but I still think it is impossible for somebody like me to have balance.

Jillian: Taylor, I think it's important to recognize that this example strikes something within you. Try not to question it – maybe play with it and take some time to think about it and then see what comes up for you.

Taylor: Maybe I will.

Jillian: I realize we have talked about some very important topics here tonight. I feel it is important that I add this in for this evening.

Up to this point we have discussed some explanations of what it means to live a balanced life. I would like to add to that and talk about something that not only I have experienced personally as an aide to creating balance in my own life, but many others also. What I am talking about here is the practice of **meditation**.

For centuries, especially within Eastern cultures, people have been using meditation as a way to cultivate a sense of serenity and balance in their lives. During the last several years, this practice has become increasingly popular amongst our modern day industrialized cultures because many of us are searching for effective ways to deal with the ever-increasing demands of our schedules. I want to introduce the concept of meditation to all of you because it can assist in the recovery process as it helps to quiet inner turmoil and despair. Many people have found that by creating the time and structure in their lives for short and simple quiet reflection, it increases their overall sense of calm and well-being.

Carly: I've done guided imagery meditation where you imagine yourself on a beach or in a peaceful place, and as you listen to the waves, you try to relax. Is this what you are talking about?

Jillian: Very similar, Carly. There are many different kinds of meditation, some more structured than others. What you are talking about sounds like a very helpful and widely used relaxation technique which is a form of meditation.

Meditation is really just the practice of being still, temporarily removing yourself from external stimulation and activity, and observing yourself for that specified period of time.

Min: Is this something we will be experimenting with during our groups?

Jillian: Min, what a wonderful idea.

Yes in fact I think now would be a wonderful time to experience meditation together.

For many years I have guided many of my group clients through a *Healing Body Meditation.* I would like to share this with all of you so you can see what it is like.

Please know that there are no *shoulds, musts, ought tos,* or *have tos* with this. The only suggestions I have for all of you are; find a comfortable place in your chair or with a pillow or blanket on the floor, close your eyes (if you would like to), and follow my voice.

This is a personal experience for each of you. You are in control at all times. If anyone becomes uncomfortable at any time during this meditation, please open your eyes and sit quietly until the others are finished with their experience.

Carly, Min, and Taylor move to the floor,
while Anika and Stephanie remain in their chairs.

Let's begin.

Take a breath in. Let your breath out. Take a few more breaths. Breathe and just take a moment to notice where you may feel your breath. Is it in your nose, with the air feeling cool going in, then warmed coming out? Do you notice your breath with the rising and falling of your chest? Or can you feel your breath in the up and down movement of your stomach? Wherever you may feel your breath, just notice it.

Take a moment and notice if you are feeling any tension or discomfort as you are noticing your breath. If you do, you can breathe into that tension, then when you exhale, let it go. Take a few moments and just follow your breath.

Today you are going on a healing journey with your body.

Your body is your sacred sanctuary. You deserve to have your entire body be nurtured and cared for. This physical body offers you so many gifts every moment each day.

Take a few breaths.

It is important to recognize that sometimes different parts of your body may serve as emotional storing houses. As you begin this healing journey with your body, please notice if any feelings come up. If they do, you do not have to do anything with them. Just follow your breath as you gently explore what is arising for you.

Notice your breath as you breathe in; notice it as you breathe out.

Notice your feet. Explore them and the way the surface may feel beneath them. Take a few breaths.

As you are focusing on your feet, notice what you are experiencing. Do you like them or hate them? Are they too big? Are your toes too fat, or are they okay? Continue to follow your breathing.

Think about what your feet have done for you over

the years, all of the places they have taken you. What kind of shoes have they worn?

Now, if you are able, see what you would like to thank your feet for: sensing the cool grass or the warm sand on the beach… Allow your feet to absorb this appreciation. Take a breath.

Would you like to apologize to your feet for anything? If so, let your feet accept your apology. How does that feel?

Now take a few breaths and move your attention to your legs.

Continue to breathe and focus on your legs, the pressure of the surface beneath them. Do you like or hate them? Are they too long or too short? Do you notice muscle and strength or do you see failure and fatigue? Follow your breath.

Think about what they have done for you over the years, how they have supported the rest of your body. What kind of clothes have they worn? What has warmed them in the winter? If your mind wanders, please bring your focus back to your breath.

See what you would like to thank your legs for: the hills they have climbed, the way they allow you to swim through bodies of water. Allow your legs to absorb this appreciation. Take a breath. Feel them absorb this.

Would you like to apologize to your legs for anything? Were you overly critical of them, or did you work them too hard? If so, let your legs absorb your apology.

Notice any sensations that may be occurring as you offer kindness to your legs.

Take a few breaths and bring your attention to your abdomen.

Do you like your abdomen or hate it? Is it comfortable or jumpy? Does it feel strong or weak? Notice if there is any discomfort. Breathe.

Think about what it has done for you over the years, how it has helped to feed and nourish you. Discover what you would like to thank your abdomen for…supporting your body with its core strength and protecting many of your internal organs. Allow your abdomen to absorb your appreciation. Take a breath and notice what this feels like.

Would you like to apologize to your abdomen? If so, let your abdomen accept your apology. Feel the release in your abdomen as you apologize.

As you take some breaths, focus your attention on your arms.

Do you like them or hate them? Are they too long or too bulky? Are you embarrassed or proud of them? Breathe into any sensations you feel.

Now for a moment, think about what they have done for you over the years, the people they have embraced, the things they have carried. Follow your breath. Notice what you would like to thank them for…opening up tactile experiences for you and helping you complete many tasks. Allow your arms to absorb your appreciations. What does this feel like?

Is there anything you want to apologize to your arms for? If so, let them accept your apology. Imagine them embracing you as you continue on.

Focus on your breathing. Notice the air coming in and the air moving out.

Bring your focus to your head. Do you like it or hate it? Does it feel well supported or would you change different features on it? Breathe.

Think about what your head has done for you over the years, the problems it has solved, the dreams and memories it holds.

In this moment is your head comfortable or is there discomfort present?

See what you would like to thank it for….allowing you to see, hear, smell, taste, talk, and think. Allow your head to absorb your appreciation. Really notice how this feels.

Continue to follow your breath.

Is there anything you want to apologize to your head for? If so, let it accept your apology.

Continue to breathe.

Take a moment now and thank your whole self for allowing you the experience of sitting quietly and embracing your mind, body, and spirit.

Follow your breath for the next few minutes. Feel it move in and out, in and out. If thoughts come, just notice them. Try not to go anywhere with them, just return to the comfort of your breathing. There will be some silence now.

As you continue into your next moments, may you carry the acceptance, kindness, and forgiveness of this meditation with you. May you continue to offer your whole being the nurturing it deserves.

Take a few minutes, and when you are ready, open your eyes, continuing to feel your breath move in and out.

Let's just sit for a moment.

When you are all able, I am wondering if anyone wants to share what this experience was like for you?

Taylor: I can't believe I actually meditated. I always thought it was some weird thing earthy crunchy people did.

It was really relaxing – in a strange way.

Jillian: I wonder if you could share with the group what felt strange.

Taylor: I've never been able to sit still for so long. I must be losing it because this felt very comforting to me.

Jillian: I don't think you are "losing it". I am glad it was comforting for you. Try to embrace this, Taylor, if you can.

I think being here in this group has allowed many of you to experiment with opening yourselves up to new experiences and new ways of thinking.

Does anybody else have any further thoughts they would like to share?

Min: I found this meditation to be very comforting. Thank you.

Jillian: You're welcome, Min.

Carly: This was very uncomfortable for me. As the meditation began I just seemed to have too many things going on in my mind.

Jillian: That sounds very challenging having to sit with so many uncomfortable thoughts.

Carly: It was!

Jillian: You made it through, Carly, even though it wasn't easy. I hope you can offer yourself something positive for that.

It is very honest and not unusual that people who are new to meditation have a similar experience. In fact, for those who have meditated for years this may still occur at times. The good thing is meditation is not about judgment of the experience and furthermore many people believe meditation can be most powerful when moments are like what you described – difficult, uncomfortable, with a wandering mind. These moments are the most beneficial when you continuously bring your mind back to your breath. For it is at these times you can sit with the difficulties without your usual reactions. This is a wonderful medium for self growth and understanding.

I want everyone to remember, you are all here experiencing new concepts and ideas about yourselves and your lives. I have a great amount of respect and admiration for each of you that continues to grow as we meet each week.

You all look quite relaxed yet tired We have experienced very intense discussions this evening. Therefore, as our time together this evening is unwinding, I will read the *Words of Hope* for all of you.

> There will be a time when we can spend the better part of our day without measuring cups. At this time, the numbers on the scale, the athletic performance, the grades on the tests, the amount of repetitions at the gym will no longer be equated with how we feel about ourselves. It is at this moment that we can really begin playing with recipes.

Before we part this evening, I want to remind all of you that we spent a great amount of time this evening discussing expectations, the ones our culture places on us and the ones we place on ourselves. This can be overwhelming and exhausting to think about. Try to offer yourselves a nurturing week.

Week Four

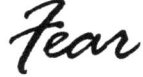

Fear

Fear is another common struggle for those who are dealing with an eating disorder. It is often fed by the underlying worry and anxiety that accompanies the actual disorder. **As humans, we have a true physiological response that occurs when we sense fear, and it directly affects our thoughts and emotions.** This healthy response may not be processed correctly in individuals with disordered thinking. In my experience when someone is entrenched in fearful thoughts, the worried mind tends to spiral out of control contributing to this feeling of fear.

Many of the girls in the eating disorder groups have explained to me that they often feel there is always a danger or catastrophe at every turn or step of the way, and therefore their life experience feels unsafe. It's as if they feel they always have a "gloom and doom" over them. What makes this more challenging for many girls is their emotional gauge in not registering correctly, as I mentioned in Week One. They often feel flooded with fear, which makes life feel more dangerous and therefore there is a greater need to protect themselves.

Many of the young women struggling with recovery rely on their obsessive behaviors to manage these feelings of fear. Some also use self injury or cutting as a way to gain control over the chaotic emotions and internal chaos. They often become attached to the temporary release of endorphins that comes with these unhealthy forms of coping. These obsessive/compulsive behaviors may deceptively offer them the comfort or safety they are craving. It often appears as if consciously or subconsciously, they are attempting to shrink away from life and all of its challenges.

I have realized when a young women is entrenched in an eating disorder she truly feels unequipped to handle the circumstances of life. Because of this, her eating disorder becomes a way of shielding herself from life and protecting herself from the challenges she feels she cannot overcome. This explains why during recovery many women express great fear over the change and unknown of not having their eating disorder to hide behind anymore.

Managing Fear

Throughout my experience in facilitating groups with young women dealing with eating disorders and body image issues, I find that using concrete strategies and tools is most effective when helping them manage their fear. For example, **visualization** and **balloon breathing** tend to tame the worried mind, calm the body, and gain control over anxiety and worried thoughts. Some young women require a **crisis plan** to help them be prepared for heightened moments of emotion. These tools can be utilized anytime and anywhere which is critical when somebody is struggling through recovery.

It is important to help young women realize that the fear is present for a reason. Through therapy and integrating new ways of coping, the fear can be examined safely and then released.

As you continue through the recovery process it is important to face your fears with the assistance of a therapist or someone you deeply trust. Often the fears you have, are created by past experiences. Talking openly about this allows your feelings of fear to become more bearable and less terrifying. Do you notice a pattern of obsessions that you think helps to minimize your fear? Or do you think the obsessions actually add to your fear? As you continue learning about yourself you will understand the purpose fear has had in protecting you and someday you will not need its destructive protection. In recovery a new fear may develop around life without your eating disorder. This is not unusual and as you read on, the group will reveal their truths about this and demonstrate hope in managing it.

> My therapist asked me if I ever think about my sister dying, and then she asked me if I was afraid of dying. But I guess I'm just afraid of living.
>
> *— Stephanie*

Jillian: Welcome to the fourth week of our group. This is actually the midway point of our nine weeks together. It seems hard to believe.

I was reflecting on this as I drove here this evening. I then began noticing the subtle changes that nature is exhibiting as the seasons shift from Winter to Spring. These changes remind me of the many shifts I see at this point in each of you.

I brought in this small tree branch with leaf buds on it to symbolize what I see occurring. Each bud is unique and is faced with its own set of challenges. Yet every bud, at its own unique time, will begin to break open and flourish into a strong, vibrant leaf, along with the promise of a new season. This tree branch reminded me of the strength I see in you, every time we meet. I do believe that each of you amazing young ladies, at your own individual times, will also have the opportunity to bloom, leaving behind all the pain and struggles that you have endured.

Thank you all for joining me here again tonight. How was everyone's week?

Carly: Before I begin, may I please sit on the floor with a pillow? I am feeling so uncomfortable today as I have all week.

Jillian: Sit wherever you are most comfortable.

Carly takes a seat on the floor, wringing her hands together.

Would you like to share what is happening right now for you?

Carly: Well, I'm really in a difficult place. I am so glad that it's finally Tuesday because I've had a really hard time, and I need to talk to someone. I have so many thoughts racing around my head right now, and I'm not sure where to begin. I'm feeling so overwhelmed. I haven't been able to sleep, and I'm feeling wired and tired at the same time. Sounds crazy, right?

Jillian: No, it doesn't sound crazy.

Is there anything that has been occurring in your life lately that may be contributing to these overwhelming thoughts and feelings you are experiencing?

Carly: My parents came up for parents' weekend. Of course, I wasn't in the swim meet because my coach won't let me compete, and I think they were really disappointed. My mother and I had a long talk about school, my eating disorder, and other deep things. She said that I looked "healthier", which is the non-offensive way of telling someone with an eating disorder they've gained weight. She said that she and my dad have been really worried about me and told me how relieved she is that I look better. I immediately felt like a fat failure. I was so angry that she said I looked "healthier". On top of that I wanted to crawl out of my own skin. I hated myself so much more. Now I feel guilty about everything that I've put them through.

Why is it so hard to just accept myself the way I am? I know I'm fatter, and I can't stand it! My stomach folds over my pants when I sit down, and I can feel my thighs rubbing together when I walk. I feel so disgusting! I am so afraid to let go of my eating disorder behaviors, because if I can't tolerate these feeling now, what will happen in the future?

Jillian: Carly, it sounds like a very challenging weekend for you. I'm glad you are here and are able to share some of the difficulties that occurred for you.

I believe it is very challenging when somebody is struggling through recovery and people offer comments about how they look, what they are eating, etc. I realize when people do this they mean it to be helpful. Yet when you are working on new thoughts and behaviors while moving away from old ones, that may have kept you feeling safe for many years, it can feel very threatening.

Week Four: Fear

I understand you are afraid to give up your eating disorder behaviors. They have allowed you to cope for many years. I am not saying that it was a healthy form of coping with your feelings, but it worked for you for that time in your life, for whatever may have been occurring. All of this can make your life feel very out of control.

If possible I wonder if you could talk a little more about what has been happening for you and how you have been able to handle all these intense emotions?

Carly: I wouldn't say I have handled anything.

I was hoping not to give in to the eating disorder behaviors – and I didn't, but I'm miserable! I don't know if I did well on my SATs, I can't swim, I'm a failure, and I can't even use exercise as an outlet. And I did something to myself that I haven't done in many years and something I promised myself I'd never do again. I cut myself. I can't believe I am crying right now, I feel so stupid. God, I am such a mess!

Carly begins to sob.

Stephanie: If it's okay, Carly, I would like to sit next to you on floor.

Stephanie joins Carly on the floor
and places her hand on Carly's back.

I'm right here if you need me.

Carly: Thank you.

Jillian: Carly, it took a lot of courage and determination on your part not to give in to the eating disorder behaviors. By doing this, you gave yourself the opportunity to feel your feelings, and this was overwhelming and painful. Try to be patient and gentle with yourself. This is an arena that is relatively new for you, and you have not yet learned to utilize alternative ways of coping with feelings.

I'm wondering if you have considered having a crisis plan so that if you ever become overwhelmed like this again, you can have a support system in place to help you get through it.

Carly: I'm not exactly sure that I know what you mean.

Stephanie: Carly, my therapist and I have worked out a plan so that I could follow specific steps if I was feeling like hurting myself. I carry people's phone numbers that I can call pretty much at any time of day if I need extra support.

Jillian: That's a really good idea. Have you found you have needed to rely on it?

Stephanie: Not very often. I think just knowing it's there gives me a lot of comfort.

Jillian: I can see how it can do that. Thank you for sharing this important information.

Carly, I wonder if you are able to take a moment and think of what your own crisis plan might look like.

Carly: I'm really not sure but I think creating a contract with myself on paper and signing it, saying that I will not cut myself and if I get to the point that I feel I need to , I will reach out to my support system.

Jillian: Carly, you have just exhibited so much strength being able to create this safety agreement for yourself. I realize this must be very difficult. It is very important that your crisis plan is something you are comfortable with and you feel you can follow through with.

Please continue to discuss this with your individual therapist, also with myself or the group if you need to.

Carly: It is so helpful for me being here tonight.

I also want to thank you for lighting that salt candle like you said you would. As I was talking tonight I would look over at it and it helped me keep on going.

Jillian: It is important that the environments you surround yourself in are comforting and helpful. If there is anything else you think could be helpful when you are here, let me know.

How is everyone else doing right now?

Taylor: I'm sorry, I just have to say something, Carly. You are so beautiful. When I saw you in the group the first night, I thought you were so pretty and smart, and I imagined that you were so popular and had no problems.

I understand what you mean about being afraid of what lies ahead and about feeling disgusting. I used to cut myself a lot when things felt really out of control – especially when my parents would fight. I used to imagine that I would punish my body for not looking the way I wanted it to. Nighttime is really hard. I hate the dark, so I always sleep with my stuffed bears and the light on and sometimes the TV. Somehow it's always helped me feel safer. There are other weird things that make me scared too. I always have someone go in the bathroom before me to see if anyone is hiding behind the curtains.

Jillian: Taylor, it sounds like you can really relate to what Carly discussed this evening.

Thank you for allowing yourself to share your struggles of fear with this group.

Taylor: No big deal.

Jillian: I wonder how you both are doing with this discussion, Min and Anika?

Min: I would like to say I guess I feel afraid for them – that they have to have these experiences in the first place.

And I feel uncomfortable to learn that Carly and Taylor would inflict pain on themselves.

I feel sadness for them.

Anika: Me, well part of me feels a sense of powerlessness – like their lives, or all of ours for that matter, is something I have no control over. And that's scary. The other part of me wants to do something to take care of them. I feel as if I have a responsibility to do so. This happens to me a lot when someone I know is in some kind of trouble.

Carly: Wait. Now I'm feeling horribly responsible for upsetting the group. Maybe I should never have said anything.

No matter what I do, it never quite feels like the right thing. I feel like I'd really like to do something to make it up to everyone. It drives me crazy how I obsess about everyone liking me and being Okay

Stephanie: I don't know if I can speak for others in the group, but I think you are amazing, Carly. Your honesty and your determination to recover is truly an inspiration.

Carly: I don't feel like much of an inspiration, I feel like a big black cloud.

Jillian: Carly, you have done nothing wrong. This is all part of the group process.

Over the past half hour, I have seen such a great amount of learning and support being exchanged between all of you in this room. Things may get difficult for others not only because of what is being said but also because of how each of us may receive it. What I mean is, people with eating disorders tend to feel not only their own pain but the pain of others around them, much more than the average person. They also tend to think they have a personal responsibility in the situation. Have any of you ever noticed that sometimes it feels as if you have distress antennas on the tops of you head? You walk around with a hyper-awareness or sensitivity to the emotions of others. You may often feel responsible for causing conflict and responsible for fixing the situation, even though it may not involve you directly. It is helpful for us all to remember that ultimately everyone is responsible for their own emotions. This can be difficult to embrace if you have, for many years, blamed yourself for the thoughts and feelings of others. It can be helpful to try to keep reminding yourselves of this and slowly you can begin to accept it.

It is not only beneficial for yourself, but also for the others here tonight that you were able to share such a difficult moment of your week with the group, Carly. I hope in sharing you will be able to heal.

If there are not any other thoughts or concerns, let's see how everyone else's week has been.

Week Four: Fear

Taylor: I'll talk about my week.

Everything's about the same, I guess. But I did remember the challenge this week because I forgot to do it the last time. For me, it was to try a new food that I haven't eaten in a while.

Jillian: How did that go for you?

Taylor: It was damn scary, but I thought about what Carly had said about how she only imagines her body is changing after she eats something scary or out of her comfort zone. It helped. I ate it a few times this week, and I'm working on ignoring the stupid eating disorder voice.

Jillian: Well done, Taylor. That sounds like a real achievement for you and you seem proud of yourself.

Taylor: Yeah, I guess for some strange reason I am. Sometimes I get sick of all the rules I live by every day.

Jillian: I hope you enjoy giving yourself some of this space to explore. I am happy for you, Taylor.

Who feels like they could share about their week next?

Min: I have done a lot of writing in my journal. I don't know if I like it, because I've been realizing some difficult things about my family. I'm so afraid they'll be disappointed in me. My grades have been slipping lately, and I'm worried about what they'll think. Grades are so important to them, especially my father. They want me to be a success. They sent me away to a good school so I could go to an elite college and then get an important job. I'm worried that my father will think I'm wasting his time and money. We have never been that close. I always felt he wanted me to be different – taller and smarter, or something. He's never been around much, always traveling. I remember when I was little I used to take his shirts out of the wash and hide them in my room because I missed him.

I was remembering all of this while I was writing, and the weirdest thing is that all I could think of was eating, eating a lot. But I didn't, and I didn't purge. I didn't give in so I could tell everyone here about it. I just kept on writing.

Jillian: I am sure this wasn't easy to do, but what a great job you did. It seems it is helpful for you, that this group is challenging you to not give into your behaviors in the same ways that you may have before we began meeting. It sounds like you were able to get through some difficult emotions in a new way. Congratulations!

Min: Thank you. I guess I was too absorbed by all the pain to view the experience in this way.

I feel a bit hopeful now.

Anika: My week has been interesting.

I had a date this week, but my parents didn't know about it because they wouldn't have approved. It was with an American boy I know from work. And I had a really good time, but now I'm so confused. I'm afraid to go against the wishes of my family with what this could all mean. They would be so angry, and they probably would make me move out. They probably wouldn't even speak to me. I'm afraid to break away from the traditions of my family, because in some ways – as restrictive as they are – they feel safe and predictable. Someone else makes decisions for you about your life.

When I noticed myself thinking about all of this, I wanted to run and hide or somehow stop the feelings. My first thought was I could eat and make it all stop, but I didn't, and now, although I feel confused and apprehensive, I feel stronger inside. I feel like I'm getting to know myself as a person separate from my family – like I'm the one in control. As overwhelming as this all feels, it's such a relief knowing I don't have to feel guilty about food.

Jillian: Anika, you bring up and interesting topic that I feel many young women can relate with.

Although you may have a desire to succeed and meet the typical developmental expectations of your age such as growing up, becoming more independent, moving away from your family, having significant friendships and relationships, going to college, or finding employment, the fear of actually attaining these things often overrides the desire. Because then what? The expectations will continue. And so, although this is not necessarily a conscious or deliberate process, many people remain entrenched in their disordered eating in order to protect themselves from the fear that accompanies moving forward.

I would like to read to you all another excerpt from the book *Gaining* by Amy Liu. I think it will fit in well with what we are talking about and hopefully explain this further.

She writes about this fear of achievement:

> It's not really fat they fear either, despite what they say. It's all those positive, powerful gains that fulfill their deeper hungers. Some tell themselves they don't deserve a lover that can make them laugh. Others fear any promotion that involves responsibility. Still others instinctively distrust anyone who befriends them. The greatest fear however, is that gaining will expose some shameful inner truth. It's not about the numbers on the scale. Deep down we all know that.

Anika: So are you saying that although it is developmentally appropriate for women our age to be seeking success and independence in our lives, for those of us struggling with eating disorders, this process gets distorted by fear.

Jillian: Yes, great job piecing this together, Anika. Let me explain this further for all of you.

Up until now we have been talking about several underlying experiences people with eating disorders have in common: overwhelming sensitivity, feelings of worthlessness, anxiety, and perfectionism, just to mention a few. If we take a closer look at all of these characteristics, it is understandable why a person with an eating disorder would want to insulate themselves from the rest of the world. To live and to experience the world as they do, life feels unsafe and threatening. The experiences other people would recognize as success, they may see potential pitfalls, because to them, achievements can trigger negative beliefs.

Anika: Would you tell us how this plays out?

Jillian: Let me think of an example to demonstrate.

Imagine you were receiving an academic scholarship and were required to attend an award ceremony with hundreds of people. To an average person, an event of this nature would most likely cause some anxiety about what one should wear, what to write for an acceptance speech, and so on. To a person with an eating disorder an occasion such as this would likely trigger enormous fear – fear not only about their physical appearance, but fear related to their moving ahead in the world, fear of being called upon to step out into center stage, to become visible. For them becoming visible means creating an opportunity where others have expectations of them. Also, it means they must have expectations of themselves. This then opens the flood gates for fear and negative thinking: "Do I really want an academic scholarship to go to college in the first place? Getting these good grades was a fluke and I'll never be able to do it again, and now everyone will expect me to. I'm a fraud, but they just do not know it yet."

Anika: I appreciate you taking the time to explain this. It makes a lot of sense to me and I have a lot to think about now.

Jillian: I'm glad it has helped you to discuss this, Anika. Stephanie, how are you doing?

Stephanie: It's kind of a funny coincidence people are talking a lot about feeling fearful and out of control, or maybe it's more than a coincidence... I made this really important discovery in therapy this week. I was talking about our group, and somehow we began talking about my sister. My therapist asked me if I ever think about her dying, and then she asked me if I was afraid of dying. But I guess I'm just more afraid of living. My mother has always had so much responsibility, and she never seems happy or has any fun. She never sits down and just relaxes. She worries about money, the house, my sister, and all of her doctor's appointments.

I guess for a lot of my life I have felt I shouldn't want things or ask for things because my mother was already so burdened. Sometimes I wish I had no desires or needs and I could just disappear. I guess, to me, the world really doesn't feel safe. It always feels like there's some kind of impending doom ahead. And sometimes I get this feeling inside that my eating disorder is the only thing that makes me feel safe, and it's so powerful it would take something far greater than it for me to recover. My therapist asked me if I ever pray. I used to believe in God, but I don't know anymore. I guess I feel pressured most of the time to figure things out on my own.

Do you think there are other ways to feel a sense of calm and safety?

Jillian: Stephanie, it sounds as if you and your therapist very effectively have been working on piecing together many thoughts and feelings about your life. It is wonderful that you have been able to share them here with us.

As for your question, yes I do know of other ways to feel a sense of calm and safety. In fact, there are several very effective ways of learning to cope with fear and overwhelming emotion. Specialists have developed many of these techniques out of their own personal struggles and need for resolution and so they could help others. Please remember, not all of them work for everyone. Many people have found they need to experiment with different ones at different times to find the right match.

Remember within our previous groups together we have talked about how powerful and consuming emotions can be. It's almost as if you become one with these feelings and they dictate how you behave. During each group we have been working on increasing awareness and sensitivity to your feelings and exploring what might be behind them. Now we will continue exploring healthier ways to regulate them.

Imagine your emotions as a car engine. I wish I could come up with a more romantic analogy. Up until now, once the engine gets going, you have had a difficult time keeping it from racing completely out of control. The strategies we will talk about will help you learn ways of slowing the engine and regaining control.

Before I present all of you with a handful of ideas, I just would like to ask, Anika: When you were speaking earlier, how it was that, although you had such a strong desire to overeat, you were able to get past these feelings without giving in to the behaviors?

Anika: Well, I know this will sound kind of ridiculous, but I didn't tell myself I couldn't eat – maybe that was wrong. I told myself to try to wait a while, and that if I really had to, I could eat later. Then, fifteen or twenty minutes would go by, and I would do the same thing. I kept doing this over and over, and pretty soon it seemed like the desire lifted or something.

Jillian: That is not silly at all. You used a very important strategy that I call **postponement**. When someone is trying to change behaviors that have become almost automatic in nature, pausing to acknowledge them, looking at the feelings or needs behind them, and then trying to delay them can be a very effective strategy. And in your case, you demonstrated that it worked!

For many people who are trying to change a behavior that is very much of an addiction, it's far too overwhelming to think of stopping for good or even for a week or an hour. That's why breaking it down into smaller, more manageable intervals of time is much more doable. And that's why in twelve step programs such as Alcoholic Anonymous or Narcotics Anonymous, members find the slogan "One Day at a Time" so helpful. Often during their recovery, they have to break it down even further –to one minute at a time.

When you're changing behaviors, it's helpful to think of the analogy of developing new muscle groups: every time you use a strategy to break unhealthy patterns, you are building and strengthening new, healthier muscles that will help your body to recover. Each time you practice using them, they will become stronger.

Another very effective way to cope with overwhelming emotions including fear is as simple as breathing. Inhaling and exhaling is something we all do, constantly, but how often do we actually stop to think about breathing. Last week when we did the meditation together, I wonder if any of you were able to realize how important and central your breathing was to that experience. In this culture, how we breathe and how our breath impacts our overall state of functioning is something rarely examined or emphasized. Once again, however, for centuries, people from Eastern countries and religions have been doing breath work to assist them with the process of meditation and relaxation. More and more, many people are looking at these practices and trying to incorporate them into their busy lives in order to reduce stress and to promote happiness and wellbeing. It is puzzling that we tend to overlook a function so vital to our livelihood and overall functioning.

Let us examine, for a moment, what happens to our bodies when we feel threatened, either physically or emotionally. Our brain sends out a message to our adrenal gland, stating there is some kind of threat. As human beings, since the beginning, this is the way we've been physiologically programmed to deal with danger. Once our adrenal gland gets the message, it begins pumping out extra adrenaline, which in turn, stimulates our heart and respiration rate. We then begin to breathe faster, our muscles tighten, our hands become clammy, and we are now physiologically prepared for fight or flight.

If you stop to consider this process more closely, it would make sense that in order to slow the body down – reverse this process – you would need to slow the breathing down. This is essentially what we are doing when we use breath work as a form of body relaxation.

Stephanie: I understand what you are saying, but could you explain how it can help when you are struggling with your eating disorder behaviors?

Jillian: I certainly can.

Many women with eating disorders, who often perceive life itself as an ever-present danger, have found if they can use breathing techniques during times of stress, they can radically reduce their unhealthy behaviors. In fact, in order to illustrate how this works and to help all of you understand further the importance of breathing, I have a guided breathing exercise which was adapted from Nancy Hopp's audio cassette **Relax, Quick**. Let's take the next few minutes and practice it together, if you feel comfortable doing so.

This breathing exercise is called **Balloon Breathing**. It is recommended that you lie on your back on a mattress or on the floor. But for us this evening, we will all be sitting upright. It is important to have your spine as straight as possible and your head and neck relaxed.

Now, if you wish, allow your eyes to close gently. Place your hand on your abdomen, just below your navel.

With the next breath you take in, direct your breath down to the bottom of your belly so when you breathe in, you can feel your hand rise when you inhale, and gently fall again when you exhale. Keep doing this for the next few minutes. Don't try to change your breath or control it, let it come naturally.

You may want to imagine there is a balloon in your abdomen, gradually inflating while you inhale, and gently deflating when you exhale. If you wish, you may even want to give the balloon a color. Really notice that color as you continue breathing.

Find a quiet, still place within you.

Keep this deep rhythmic flow going.

Let yourself be captured by this natural flow.

Within each inhale as the balloon inflates, you may want to imagine yourself breathing in calm and peace, and with each exhale, as the balloon deflates breathing out stress and fear. Enjoy how this may feel.

> Begin to notice there is a quiet centered place
> within yourself, so that anytime and anywhere there
> is distraction and external noise, you can return to this
> place of calm.
>
> When each of you feels ready and are able, you can
> begin wiggling your toes, moving your hands, and
> finally open your eyes.

I would like you to know how brave I think you all are. Each and every one of you showed great trust in me and yourselves to try this exercise.

Would anyone like to share how this was for them?

Carly: I know I've taken up a lot of this group tonight, but I really enjoyed this.

After all my own personal drama, I have to say I feel like I have slowed down for a few moments and for once I'm not afraid of that.

Min: I can relate, Carly.

As we were breathing, I felt as if my shoulders became lighter. It was like for a few moments, all the deep and painful emotions that have been coming up for me, were somehow lessened.

Jillian: I am thrilled that the both of you were able to experience how a breathing exercise like this can help give you a break from all the discomfort you are experiencing within the moments of your days.

Another comforting thought about using breathing when fear arises is that this technique is portable. You can take it with you and use it just about anywhere and at any time.

I would like to discuss another effective technique that may be helpful to each of you when you are feeling stressed or overwhelmed. This technique is called **visualization**.

Our imagination is also a very powerful tool. And just as our seeing an image of a distressing situation can make us feel uncomfortable and tense, imagining something warm, safe, secure, and positive can make us feel more relaxed. When we are in a situation where our fear is racing out of control, another way to help us regain composure and calm is to imagine we are part of a peaceful scene. We can also utilize this technique while we are slowing down our breathing.

Stephanie: I think visualization sounds very difficult if I am already feeling out of control in my thought and feelings.

Jillian: Great point. I can explain how to deal with this in greater detail.

People have found it is easier to construct what this scene would look like ahead of time, rather than trying to create it while they are in the middle of a crisis. This way, the scene is readily available if and when it is needed. All that is required is for you to imagine a place of total comfort and safety, a place you have experienced at some point in your lives. If you cannot remember one, just imagine one. Recall, or imagine the sights, smells, sounds, and sensations that accompany this place. Remember how your body felt (or would feel) being there. Imagine what you might have been thinking (or what you would be thinking) if you were really there. Imagine being there. This is your peaceful place. You will be able to return to this place anytime you need to feel safe.

Stephanie: That sounds too good to be true – but very interesting. I never thought of doing something like this to help me when I am struggling.

Jillian: Stephanie, I think it is important to acknowledge, that for you, our discussion has stretched your thinking a bit. This can be very positive and helpful.

I want to offer all of you girls many tools to help you on your journey of recovery. Use whatever feels right to you whenever you may need. Play with these techniques, be creative and make them yours.

It is wonderful how many of you seem able to identify with some of these techniques. Therefore, I would like to continue offering you a few other skills that can help each of you, when coping with fear or any other challenging feelings or thoughts.

Another technique, that I have often used to help the girls in my groups when they struggle with fear of change and the unknown, etc, is called **anchoring**. I have adapted this technique from Mark Thornton's audio cassette *Meditation in a New York City Minute*: *Super Calm for the Super Busy*. With this technique, you can actually create emotional states you feel you are lacking in. You can create the feeling of calm, strength, confidence, or whatever feelings a situation might call for. This technique involves two stages. The first stage is called **Building the Anchor** and the second is **Firing up the Anchor**.

Here's how it works.

If you were in a need of strength, you do the following:

First you would build the anchor. The process begins by closing your eyes. Remembering a time when you felt especially strong, just the way you would like to feel right now. Ask yourself the following questions. What was it like for you to feel this way? How was your breath? How was your tone of voice? How did your body feel? What did people say about you? Then it is time to build up this feeling of strength inside of you – spreading it around throughout your body. This is done by putting your thumb and forefinger together, creating an anchor for this feeling.

Now, firing up the anchor can occur whenever you are in a situation that calls for strength, by placing your thumb and forefinger together to recall these feelings.

You can use this technique to create other feeling states by following the same format.

Does anybody have any questions or comments?

Nobody is saying anything, and you all look very focused listening, so I would like to continue on with one last one.

Now I would like to discuss one of my personal favorite techniques for dealing with overwhelming emotions. This is **mindfulness**. Today there's a lot of talk about the concept of mindfulness. It's actually a meditation and a philosophy that is deeply rooted in the ancient principles of Tibetan Buddhism. When we practice being mindful, we make a conscious decision to try to be totally present or aware of this very moment in time – where we are, how we are, who we're with, the sights and smells around us, the feelings we have at the present time – but without any judgment about our experience.

Taylor: This mindfulness stuff freaks me out. Why would I want to be so deeply in each moment when I can't stand so much of what happens in my soap opera style life?

Jillian: You raise an interesting question. Taylor.

Basically the skill of mindfulness is looking at your feelings from a vantage point which is more distant and less overwhelming, so that you can experience your feelings without being engulfed by them. However, an important component here that I have not discussed before is when you observe your feelings with a mindful stance, it is important to do so without judging them.

Perhaps the best way to get this point across is to give you an example of how someone with an eating disorder might put this into practice.

I would like to ask you all to take this time to pause and just relax in the silence as I read to you a *Vignette on Mindfulness*. I believe this will help you all understand this concept a little more clearly.

Jenn was home alone after a long and frustrating day at school. The girls at school seemed more flirtatious and gossipy then usual and the boys more immature. Jenn thought of the afternoon of homework she had in front of her and could think of nothing else except checking out the cupboards in the kitchen and examining the remaining leftovers from last night's dinner. She really didn't want to think about avoiding a binge, utilizing coping skills, or having to tell the whole world about wanting to binge. She became angry, resentful, and despairing. She thought, "Why can't life just be simpler?"

She mustered up whatever strength she had and decided to take a walk to the bridge nearby, where she and her sister used to watch sticks float down the river. She reluctantly decided to try the mindfulness activity she had previously learned about in the group. She imagined her thoughts and feelings sitting on top of the water, drifting down stream like pieces of wood. She observed and described with as little judgment or criticism as possible.

First, she noticed feeling really hyper and said, "That's a hyper feeling floating by."

She began feeling really self conscious and stupid about what she was doing, but she just watched curiously as those feelings went by. As she stayed and watched her emotions, she neither tried to hold onto them nor push them away. She observed everything and labeled them as thoughts, feelings, or emotions. She noticed many thoughts about wanting to eat and to return home.

Over time, she started to observe and experience a sensation of sadness and disappointment in her throat and chest. She stayed and watched them go by. Although it wasn't all pleasant, she slowly observed a feeling of warmth and calmness approaching as she continued with the exercise.

After about twenty minutes had passed, she noticed the sun was setting and thought she should be on her way. Jenn stopped at a friend's house on her way home, visited for awhile, and made it through the day without bingeing.

Taylor: Does mindfulness only help with bingeing?

Jillian: No, Taylor. Let me explain more.
The skill of mindfulness can also be applied to the discomfort that comes with having to eat, for those who are used to restricting, or the bloated feeling that can come from following

a meal plan. Essentially, the same technique is used – observing without judging – and it can be used any time feelings are overwhelming or distressing. In fact, mindfulness can help heal a person's dysfunctional relationship with food and create a healthy balance through a practice called **mindful eating**.

Mindful eating is simply applying the same basic principle of awareness to eating. We spend so much of our lives being in a hurry and trying to capitalize on our use of time. It is rare that people only do one thing at a time, and even rarer to give whatever we're doing our fullest attention. We talk on the phone while we drive. We watch television while we eat. We problem solve while we fall asleep at night or upon waking. It is rare to be totally in the present. Increasingly, people who are conscious of wanting to live a healthier and more meaningful life are practicing mindful meals.

Stephanie: For the life of me, I cannot imagine what that would be like.

Jillian: Does anyone have any thoughts?

Anika: I think it is being quiet and conscious of what you're eating.

Jillian: Absolutely, Anika. But it goes beyond that, by first being very mindful of how your body feels before you eat. Then examine how hungry you are. Is your stomach growling? Are you getting lightheaded? Are you anxious?

Many people sit down to a meal in a setting where they know there aren't any distractions, and that way, when they begin to eat, they are fully aware, conscious of the textures of the food, the sweetness or saltiness, how it feels inside their mouth when swallowing it, and so on. They pay careful attention to how their body feels once it has eaten. Is it satisfied or does it want more? How full does it feel?

Anika: People do this every time they eat?

Jillian: They strive to. Of course, it's not always feasible, given the fact that we do live such busy lives, but even if you can just practice this whenever you have an opportunity, it will slowly influence your overall eating patterns.

Anika: This all seems very uplifting yet uncertain to imagine living my life with curiosity for my feelings without judgment, while allowing myself to create enough space to be aware of what is happening moment to moment for me.

Jillian: Very well said, Anika. I think it is wonderful that you can look ahead yet be aware that some doubt still remains. This thought of yours reminds me of something I like to call **creating a climate for change**.

I realize I have given you all a lot of information on how to begin making changes in your lives, and I want to reiterate that change doesn't happen all at once. It is a gradual process, and different coping strategies work for different people. However, I have found that various factors or circumstances can either support or inhibit a person's efforts to change. Therefore, I feel it will be useful to explore this for a moment.

Please try to imagine your eating disorder to be a life raft, there to help keep you afloat in a tumultuous sea. What are some of the factors you would need to make it possible for you to let go of the raft? What would you require to be able to trust that you would be Okay? Knowing what some of these factors are can help you to be proactive in creating an environment conducive to change.

Let's do this for a moment. In no particular order, just verbalize what each of you thinks would be helpful for you.

Carly: For me, I would need someone else to be by my side, so I could tell them repeatedly how scared I was.

Stephanie: I'd need people to understand what I was going through.

Anika: I would need to tell myself that whatever I was feeling, it would be temporary. Also, it would help for others to remind me it was only temporary.

Stephanie: I would also need unconditional love, acceptance, companionship, and reassurance.

Min: Reasonable expectations, from myself and others would help me.

Carly: I think it would be helpful to keep my healthy goals closely in sight, like written everywhere or something.

Anika: Distraction, relaxation, structure.

Stephanie: The reassurance I was getting from others would have to be stronger and louder than my own self-doubts.

Taylor: Maybe an inpatient or residential setting, someone else to take control if I couldn't let go.

Min: Faith.

Jillian: Bravo to all of you. I hope you all realize how hard each of you has worked here this evening. This work is difficult. I think it is very admirable that you come here every Tuesday with the ability to share, listen, and support.

Does anybody have any questions or comments about anything we have discussed this evening?

I think now is a great time to read to you all our *Words of Hope* for this evening. Sit back and receive this thought in the way that is most helpful for you.

> Fear develops because we have learned to associate certain experiences with painful and intolerable reactions. When we discover we have the resources to deal with these overwhelming feelings, either found within us or in the connection we make with others, we are free to dream of the future.

As we end our time together this evening, I wish you all a hopeful week. Be well. See you next time.

Week Five

Control

For young women dealing with eating disorders, the issue of **control** is a true struggle. Many often feel they are in a constantly vulnerable place, falling prey to life's unpredictable and potentially harmful terms. It is as if they feel a sense of disempowerment.

What complicates this even further is that these girls lack protective boundaries for themselves. They do not have boundaries around their own negative self talk or the many expectations they may have for themselves. For many, there is also a lack of boundaries with people in their world. It is known that there is a relationship between uncomfortable situations and negative body image. For example, when a person has an eating disorder and their boundaries are violated, they may immediately think "I've gained weight".

Many of these young women use obsessive behaviors around food and exercise in an attempt to experience the world in a more predictable way. The voice of the eating disorder (as mentioned in Week 2) can convince them that in being faithful to their disorder they are in control, when in reality it is the eating disorder that is adding to the loss of control. While intending to manage their inner and external chaos with these eating disorder behaviors, more chaos is actually created.

Managing Control

As the process of recovery evolves, the following skills can be helpful in managing this issue of control: **creating healthy boundaries, setting realistic expectations, assertive communication, and identifying triggering situations.**

Oftentimes it has been my experience that due to the biochemical imbalance that is prevalent, it may become necessary to utilize medication as a way to regulate the imbalance and aide in regaining a sense of healthy control. **Medication is useful in relieving anxiety, depression, and the heightened sensations of their emotions.** Combined with behavioral approaches and therapy, this has offered many positive results.

During recover with the combination of modalities, many of these young women are able to discover that they cannot control circumstances or other people's thoughts, feelings, or behaviors. They are often empowered by the realization that what they actually do have control of is their own response and reaction. Eventually this begins to feel very liberating.

As you learn about the purpose your eating disorder may be serving, I wonder if you have thought about in what circumstances, or with whom in your life, you feel a loss of control. Throughout your recovery you will begin to discover new and healthy ways that allow you to have a sense of healthy balance in your life, regardless of what may be happening around you. These new skills are not only helpful in eating disorder recovery, but can be beneficial in future situations and relationships. As you will witness in the group, it can be challenging trying on these new ways of coping with the issue of control, even awkward. Trust in yourself and your newly developing abilities, to handle these intense thoughts and feelings in ways that can offer you the security you are craving.

They argued for what felt like hours. I went up to
my room, but I felt so trapped up there. My body felt
disgusting and I couldn't think of anything else.

– Taylor

Jillian: Hello to all of you.

As we gather together again, I wonder how all of you are
doing. We have discussed many suggestions of how to better
cope with the challenges that go on with an eating disorder.
I recognize that this might all feel a little overwhelming, so I
thought we could have a brief *Coping Skill Review*. I realize
this sounds scholastic, I promise it is not, but I feel it can be
very helpful. This way if you are in a stressful situation and feel
yourself being pulled to use unhealthy behaviors, you may feel
more familiar with, and be able to decide which coping skill
might be the most useful to you.

> *Stephanie appears anxious as she*
> *repeatedly looks towards the door.*

Stephanie: I don't mean to interrupt, but is Taylor not coming
this evening?

Jillian: I have not heard from her at all, Stephanie. Are you feeling concerned?

Stephanie: Yes, I guess I am. It feels strange to me to be missing
one person in the group, it is not like it usually is.
I hope she is okay.

Jillian: I completely understand your concern, Stephanie. It is
only ten minutes after six. Maybe she will arrive shortly. If not
I will try to follow up with her. In the meantime, while we are
waiting, let's begin reviewing the coping skills.
I decided to summarize what we have discussed because
up to this time we have discussed a great amount. The way I

would like to do this is to have all of you listen, however you are comfortable, as I discuss each one briefly. Please ask any questions if you need to.

I will begin with **Positive Self Talk**. This is learning to talk to yourself in a kind and nurturing voice, in order to counter the harsh shaming voice. Imagine yourself using the same compassionate tone you would use with a child.

Next, **Radical Acceptance** is a way to approach yourself and your situation with two wings – a wing of wisdom or seeing and a wing of compassion. You need two wings to fly.

Affirmations are wonderfully effective. These are supportive and nurturing words or phrases, composed in advance, which can be recited during stressful times.

Another is **Rainbow Thinking**. This way of thinking challenges you to view the world in more than black and white. This perception may help you to set expectations for yourself and others which are more reasonable.

Self Nurturance is simply caring for yourself by paying attention to your underlying needs, and then to try to satisfy them in ways that are caring and nourishing.

Meditation is the concept of adapting a quiet, peaceful, and contemplative stance. It is used for relaxation and to restore a state of equilibrium when feeling anxious and overwhelmed.

Breathing is using breath work to help you achieve a state of calm and wellbeing. This can be used anywhere and anytime. Breathe in a feeling of peace and calm, breathe out stress and fear.

Visualization involves using your imagination to assist you in visualizing a calm, safe place that can hold you during stressful times. This technique can be used to help calm you when you are overwhelmed by uncomfortable emotions.

Anchoring promotes or enhances feelings of calm, courage, or confidence by using visualization to imagine a time when these feelings were previously experienced, then placing your thumb and forefinger together to create and anchor.

Finally, **Mindfulness** means observing with full attention, with curiosity, and without judgment. This can be very helpful when used to create distance from overwhelming emotions. It can also be used to promote self-acceptance and reduce feelings of worthlessness and shame.

I hope this was helpful for you all and not more confusing.

I wonder what some of you were thinking or feeling as I read these to you?

Min: I didn't find it confusing at all. In fact it helped me piece together all that we have been discussing.

It seems clearer to me that I have options beyond all this disordered eating of mine.

Carly: I have to say I enjoyed this very much. As you were speaking, I felt a little like I used to when my parents would read to me when I was young. I know that sounds weird, but I really liked hearing these coping skills being stated out loud.

Jillian: It doesn't sound strange. I think something in you craves this kindness and compassion for yourself. When you were younger and you may have been snuggled in your bed listening to your favorite story, I am guessing you felt very loved, safe, and cared about. For many years these comfortable feelings have been shadowed by an eating disorder. So, I am glad listening to the coping skills offered you something so pleasant.

And, Min, I think it is wonderful for you that these coping skills may be offering you new ways of handling your life.

Are there any other comments or questions?

Taylor bursts into the room

Taylor: Oh my god, I am such a loser!

I am sorry for being so late and crashing through the door like that.

My life is really falling apart. I hope it is okay that I am here.

Jillian: Please, Taylor, sit down, and take a few slow breaths. We are glad you were able to make it here this evening. Would you like to share with us what has been going on?

Taylor: Things aren't going that well for me. Friday night my dad got really drunk, and my parents were fighting about money. There was a lot of yelling and furniture flying everywhere. It was worse than usual. Our neighbors called the police, and my idiot dad got arrested and spent the night in jail. And now my parents aren't talking to each other, and they're not talking to our neighbors because they called the cops.

So I was really upset on Friday. I wasn't feeling that well to begin with. My stomach hurt, and I was resting on the couch when it all started. They argued for what felt like hours, so I eventually went up to my room. I felt so trapped up there. I had nowhere to go. I tried drowning out the noise by watching TV but it didn't help. I wanted to leave the house, but I had nowhere to go.

My body felt disgusting, and I couldn't think of anything else. I hated everything about it. I felt dirty and gross, and I kept hearing the words "You're so fat and stupid" over and over. "You're so weak for giving in and trying to get better. You can't do anything right, and you'll never change!" I knew it was the eating disorder voice, but no matter what I did, I couldn't stop it. So I stayed in my room all night and actually most of the weekend. I relapsed into my old ways of depriving myself of just about anything good for me. What scares me is it felt really good in a lot of ways. I felt empty and clean and numb to everything around me. I forgot how good it felt.

I'm really worried because I don't want to slip back completely. I don't want to go back to the freakin hospital.

Jillian: I'm sorry you had to be in the middle of a situation where you felt so alone and desperate, where you felt there was nothing you could do, Taylor. If you can, try to be easy on yourself and find some compassion for yourself. You are learning new skills, so eventually you can make healthier choices, but remember, recovery is a process which does not occur overnight. The fact that you even considered looking behind the eating disorder voice for something else you might be feeling or needing is great progress. Your eating disorder has been in your life for a long time, and it takes time and practice to learn new ways to deal with situations, especially those which evoke such pain.

Carly: Taylor, I don't mean to interrupt, but the fact that you are here tonight and you're talking about what happened is really good. It shows how strong you are and how much you really do want to recover. I guess it can be really hard when you start making changes, but the world around you is still staying the same.

You know my therapist always tell me there's a difference between a lapse and a relapse, and if you get back on track quickly, it's just a lapse, not a complete relapse. She says the longer you let yourself slip back, the harder it is to turn it around. So maybe you can just think of this as a lapse.

It's often hard for me to imagine living with the amount of chaos you have in your life. Things must feel so scary and out of control.

Taylor: Thanks, I wish I could see this the way you do – I am not a very positive person. And yes, my life does suck – it always has.

Jillian: Taylor, do you think your parents know how all of this affects you?

Taylor: I think my mother knows something's up because she keeps asking me what I've had to eat, or maybe she just feels guilty or something. It drives me crazy when she does this. She thinks I'm a two-year old. It just gets me that much angrier, and when I'm that angry, I want to starve just to get back.

Jillian: Taylor, I respect all that you have just said and I can understand it. For years, your eating disorder may have offered you a false sense of control when people and situations around you may have felt out of control. Feeling out of control can be very scary and overwhelming, so it does make sense that you want to control something.

Taylor, you are not alone. In the years of facilitating these groups, I have learned that the majority of women struggling with an eating disorder have held fast to an underlying belief that their eating disorder had something to do with control. They may not have been exactly certain how this factor was related to their disorder, but they speculated there was a connection of some kind.

For one moment, let's all try to think about this a little further. I'm wondering if any of you are able to see the role fear, anxiety, and chaos – whether internal or external – play in your lives? Can you see how your eating disorder has led you to believe it has been a viable solution to your problems?

Stephanie: Yes I can. It can almost feel like a friend who then quickly and quietly becomes your worst enemy. Yeah, maybe for a while things feel clearer and less complicated. You feel like you have a mini supply of safety, security, and confidence, but then it begins to take over your whole life, and you can't think of anything else. You find yourself getting angry at everything, for no apparent reason. The people and activities which were at one time special no longer matter anymore. Everything starts feeling foggy and complicated again.

Taylor: Yeah, I know what you mean, Stephanie.

Jillian, I don't know if this is what you are talking about. I've been told I have attention issues, but you know earlier how you said to look behind your negative body thoughts to see what you're really feeling about a situation? Well, I tried to do that the other night. I felt badly enough about what was going on in the house as it was. I didn't want to have all of those disgusting feelings about my body on top of it. So I tried to separate them, but I just couldn't. Each time I tried to think about what was happening at home, I felt too scared and shaky. I'm so angry at myself for giving into my old crappy behaviors.

Jillian: Taylor, what a well stated explanation and example of what can occur when we are bombarded by fear, anxiety, and chaos. Please be gentle with yourself. Even though you may have given in to old behaviors, your thoughts were different. You were attempting to explore new ways to experience your feelings in this difficult situation. Every time you do this, the healthier part of you is becoming stronger. This does sound like an extremely scary and overwhelming situation you experienced, and the fact that you were able to do this exploring demonstrates great strength from within you. I feel grateful that you have come here tonight and were able to share so much of your experience.

I wonder if it feels helpful to you?

Taylor: I guess a little. I mean talking about it does make me feel like I'm not so trapped by this crappy experience. Being here is always nice. It's the only place right now where I don't feel judged. I guess being here, is kind of like having a stable family compared to the crazy family I have at home.

Jillian: Thank you for sharing, Taylor.

I wonder how everyone else is doing?

Min: I have to say something. I had no idea what I was getting myself into when I started all this. I just wanted to lose weight. I didn't know it could be so dangerous. I understand now why everyone around me made such a big deal out of it when they found out. I guess I'm not the only one with problems.

Jillian: So are you saying that you are learning a lot about yourself by being a part of the group?

Min: Yes, definitely. I find it difficult sometimes listening to all the pain we share, but mostly I find it helpful because I don't feel so isolated. It has been very difficult at times living in a different culture without my family. When I come to our group I am not only figuring things out, but also feeling connections that I haven't felt in many years.

Jillian: It is meaningful that you have allowed us into your life, Min. All of you girls bring something special to our coming together.

Anika: I have been trying to practice the mindfulness skill and to continue writing in my journal. And it seems to be working, because my eating has been so much better.

My family was definitely into my business this week. They still don't know about my date with an American boy, but my aunt and my mother had a recent conversation about my eating and commented on how there seemed to be more food remaining in the house. This got me so angry. When they're in my business, I feel so out of control! I definitely felt like I wanted to lose it – and eat – and take all the frustration out on myself, but I tried the mindfulness exercise. First, I began to practice deep breathing, and then I imagined I was stepping outside myself to observe what was happening. What was the emotion? Well, I was angry and frustrated. How was it making me feel? That was easy. Like a child without any respect. I didn't judge myself for feeling this way. I kept breathing deeply and slowly, and eventually the panicky and angry feelings seemed to pass. I know it must all sound kind of weird. But I didn't eat, and then I wrote about it. I feel so much stronger for not giving in to the unhealthy behaviors.

Jillian: Anika, it sounds like you did a great job of practicing to nurture yourself instead of giving into old unhealthy patterns. Well done! Sometimes when you do this it feels like you're doing the exact opposite of what you really want to do at the time.

Anika: That is absolutely true, but I am so sick of my life being ruled by food the way it is.

Jillian: Great point. Many young girls who are in recovery come to a point where their eating disorder does not satisfy them the way it used to. This can be a seed for change to occur.

Anika, it sounds like you and your family may struggle with having healthy boundaries. I would like for a moment to explain to you all the notion of **boundaries** and how they may affect many of your behaviors.

As humans, we construct certain parameters around us, sometimes visible and sometimes not, which help us create a corral of personal safety and comfort. This structure helps us to maintain a sense of privacy from others when we do not want them to know personal details about us, and it helps us to maintain a healthy distance from people we choose not to become emotionally close to. There are times when we need to create boundaries even with those people we love and care about, as in those instances we may need to close a bedroom door or ignore a telephone call. Often, it is when the boundaries we've constructed have been violated by others that we are left feeling unprotected, frightened, and out of control. These overwhelming feelings can then lead us to engage in unhealthy behaviors as a way of coping with the intrusion or violation.

Anika: This is definitely what happens for me. So what can be a solution?

Jillian: Perhaps one way to deal with this would be to try to begin noticing areas of your life where you feel someone has crossed your boundaries and to consider whether there is an effective way of communicating this to that person.

Anika: That sounds easy, but I'm not sure I will be effective at communicating things to others – I've never been very assertive.

Jillian: Developing healthy forms of communication is all part of this process. It begins with communicating with yourself and then this will develop into feeling comfortable with asserting yourself to others.

Anika, it sounds like you are learning to assert yourself through journaling. Try to be as patient with yourself as you can.

Anika: Thanks, I will.

Jillian: Is there anyone else who would like to share what has been happening for them?

Carly: There is something I've had on my mind and I was wondering if I could bring it up.

Jillian: Certainly, please do.

Carly: Okay We've been talking a lot lately about anxiety, so I've been doing a lot of thinking about how much worrying I do about being perfect at everything and how I have mood swings and, if things get out of hand, I can even have a panic attack and can't breathe. Well, I've been talking with my therapist about possibly being evaluated for medication. But the thing is, I'm worried it will make me not care anymore – about any-thing – and I'm worried about gaining weight. In some ways, I really like caring so much about issues in the world. What if I end up like a zombie? Or what if I start gaining weight and I don't even realize it?

Stephanie: Carly, I started taking medication around the time the group started, and I had so many of the same concerns. My therapist tried to get me to consider being evaluated years ago, but I just wasn't ready. I'm really beginning to see it making a difference in how much obsessing I'm doing about things, and I think I have more energy, in general. I don't feel so spacey, and it's easier to get work done. I'm on a really low dose to start out.

Carly: I'm just so freaked out by the idea of it. Maybe it won't work the same for me.

Jillian: Carly, I can understand your concerns about medication. It's a very difficult decision to make. However, for many people with eating disorders, it has made recovery for them so much easier. For others, it has even saved their lives. People some-times get stuck in their unhealthy thinking and behaviors be-cause of an underlying chemical imbalance. For these people, when the anxiety or depression is more manageable, it is easier for them to move forward in recovery.

I would like you all to know it can sometimes take a while to find the right medication or the right dosage, again this is a process. The most common medications used for eating disorders are called antidepressants. They can help balance the chemicals in your brain, so your body can begin to re-lease more of the "feel good" chemicals. These chemicals not only improve your mood but they also help slow down your thoughts and therefore allow room for you to explore your feelings and needs more clearly.

Carly: What if the medication changes who I am?

Jillian: Your concerns are very real. I want to assure you that medication does not overpower you and you will not become controlled by it.

The medication actually allows you more opportunity to gain healthy control over your thoughts and behaviors. This can be very helpful in actually allowing yourself to be more of who you really are on many levels.

Carly: I am so scared I will have to take it forever to be okay.

Jillian: Another great point. It is scary to wonder if you will need medication for your entire life.

Carly, let me remind you to try to focus on what you need for this time in your life. Try not letting yourself get too far ahead – although I know this is easier said than done. Generally when someone begins taking medication to help with their eating disorder struggles, they are not on it for years and years.

Maybe this will help. Think of when somebody becomes injured when playing sports. The athletic trainer may work with the person to strengthen the injured part and make it stronger alongside the physician who may have prescribed some muscle relaxants and pain medicine. Together these two techniques aide the healing of the injury and allow the athlete to prevail, hopefully stronger and more balanced in the area of the injury than before. Once the athlete is over this "hump" of their recovery process, the medicine is no longer needed.

This would more than likely be the same for you, Carly, or any of you girls. The medication, along with therapy can aide in getting you over the difficult humps in your recovery. Then when you are at a stronger, more balanced place in your recovery process (and you will know when), the medicine may no longer be necessary.

Carly: I guess I never thought of it like that. Thank you for taking the time to explain this.

Jillian: You're welcome. This is a very important piece of recovery and I am glad it was brought up.

Carly, I would like to advise you to consider continuing to discuss your fears and concerns with your therapist and parents. In doing so you may come to a time when it will be easier for you to consider trying medication, if it is necessary.

Carly: I can do that. I do think it can help.

Jillian: Does anyone have anything else they want to share?

Stephanie: I would like to tell the group about my experience. I had wanted to try the visualization exercise, and I did. I really enjoyed doing it.

I wanted to share it with all of you. Can I read you my visualization of my safe place?

Jillian: I think that would be very nice to hear.

Stephanie reaches into her back pack
and takes out a piece of notebook paper.

Stephanie: I hope this sounds okay?!

I'm a little girl, and its Thanksgiving, and my family and I are going to my grandmother's house, where all of my favorite cousins are. There is an abundance of delicious smells in the house and festivity filling the air. There are little baskets of treats at every place setting with our names on them. It's warm and safe, and there's a music box down the hall that I can't wait to play with after dinner. We watch movies and play board games, and because it's too far to drive home at night, we get to sleep over on light blue sheets that smell of sweet laundry soap. And then I imagine being in the arms of my grandmother.

I don't know if you can see it, but I'm wearing a charm around my neck of a music box so that when I feel scared I can hold it in my hand. Having it so close to me reminds me that my safe place isn't so very far away.

Jillian: It is very encouraging that you enjoyed creating this visualization. I hope you will find it helpful when you encounter some struggles.

Week Five: Control

Stephanie: I do think I will. I mean, even as I read this to all of you, I am experiencing what I am saying with all of my senses. It is strange but also very comforting.

Taylor: It must be nice to have an actual place like this that you can think of. I haven't got that. I may need to borrow yours because it sounds so nice to me. I wish I was there this past weekend!

Stephanie: My safe place can be your safe place if you need it to be.

Taylor: That's really cool of you.

Jillian: Stephanie, you were really able to capture the elements with your visualization that create a sense of peace for you. It is wonderful that you can still connect so deeply to this experience at your grandmother's house.

One thing I would like you all to remember, like we discussed last week, even if you cannot think of or remember a time or place that you felt best; it is just as effective to imagine one. Stephanie, thank you for sharing this with our group.

Stephanie: I am glad I have such special people around me.

Jillian: This evening has involved a lot of important discussion for a many of you. Much of what we have talked about tonight is connected to **control**. I think is important for us to investigate this idea of control and talk a little about finding healthy control.

Min: I do not mean to interrupt, but why is control so important to us as human beings?

Jillian: Great question! I believe if each of you stop and really think about the meaning behind the word "control", you can see just why it's so important in our lives. We need to feel we are able to have an impact over our lives and to be able to somehow influence the course of events that affects each one of us and our loved ones. If we had no ability to do so, we

would be lost. Someone or something else would be completely navigating our everyday activities, their outcomes, and the
bigger plans for our destiny.

Carly: This sounds like control that everyone strives for. Then
why is it that my therapist is always trying to explain to my
parents about my eating disorder and how I use it to feel in
control.
    I guess I understand it, but not clearly.

Jillian: Well, many psychologists believe people with eating
disorders adopt unhealthy behaviors around food and weight
as a way of compensating for circumstances in life they feel
they have little or no control over. The eating disorder becomes
one area of control in the midst of chaos and change. In many
ways, this is a really logical solution. However, as we all are
well aware, it is also one that can become self-destructive and
dangerous.

Carly: This is clearer. I guess when I heard my therapist use the
word control, it would feel like people were judging me as a
controlling person. When now I understand it has been a way
for me to survive.

Jillian: Absolutely. I want to invite you all to consider an alternative way of looking at control: **What if the pursuit of a healthy,
balanced, and self-nurturing life could be where you could
exercise your control? What if, in the midst of chaos and turmoil, your quest for stability, inner strength, and equilibrium
could be your means of gaining control?** This would mean
making a commitment to practice, not to perfection. It would
mean practicing with a healthy, well-balanced diet, getting a
moderate amount of exercise, and, in keeping with the tenets
of the Live-It, caring for your mental, physical, emotional, and
spiritual selves.

Carly: This sounds too good to be true. Right now it seems this
would work for others, but not for me. It is too overwhelming

and scary to imagine facing this world without the rules I have created for myself.

Stephanie: I agree with what you are saying, Carly. For me, some days I feel stronger and seem able to face challenges with healthier choices. But other days, watch out, if I bend any of my rules I feel like I am going to fall to pieces.

Jillian: This is why I would like you all to just become a little bit curious about the choices that healthy control involves and find some power in this. For example, when Anika's family made comments about the food that had remained in the cabinets longer than it had previously, she felt personally violated – understandable so.

Anika, is this the type of situation that you found to be difficult for you?

Anika: Yes, yes.

Jillian: Well, had she chosen not to utilize her newly learned skills, she could have easily ended up bingeing. This was truly a **triggering situation**, a situation which set in motion feelings and thoughts that could easily have led to unhealthy actions. Anika made a choice to find a healthy control versus unhealthy control.

Min: But this is difficult to do when you are in the middle of a hard time.

Jillian: Yes it is. This is why I believe that developing a concrete plan for emotional crisis, meltdowns, or setbacks can have a great impact over one's well being. In doing so, even the unexpected or unmanageable could be made to feel more manageable.

Carly: I know we talked about some of this last week, but could you tell me a little more about how this actually works.

Jillian: Sure. This can be accomplished by developing a crisis plan and drawing from the many strategies we have covered in our groups. It is also important to become familiar with the specific situations that typically trigger overwhelming reactions, because then you can be better prepared for them – or they can all together be avoided. What I often tell many of the girls in my groups is to make a list of situations in their life that are particularly triggering. Then, right next to the list, write down ways they could manage them effectively if they were in a triggering situation.

Carly: I can see how this can help.

Min: This makes sense, yet it doesn't. What I mean is, if we take healthier control of our lives, there is still so much we cannot control. It's all still about control. Sometimes it seems like too much.

Jillian: It can be. This is when I like to use the idea of **letting go**.

Just think of this for a minute. I have encouraged you all to take more control over your lives by taking healthier steps to care for yourselves, now I'm going to introduce an approach that will probably seem like a complete contradiction.

I wonder if any of you are familiar with the serenity prayer which is often read in twelve step programs such as Alcoholics Anonymous or Narcotics Anonymous: "God, grant me the serenity to accept the things I cannot change, the courage to change the things I can, and the wisdom to know the difference." It is a prayer or a philosophy widely practiced in recovery programs. People who are fighting addictions find it useful because they have difficulty recognizing and accepting there are often challenging situations in their lives they have little control over. It reminds them they have an inner strength which can help them get through challenging situations without resorting to unhealthy patterns. It also suggests to them there are other sources of strength available to them, if they need it, for those situations that warrant additional support. This may come in the form of some kind of spiritual guidance or just support from other program members. The concept is truly just about realizing that there are an awful lot of things in life that we do have control over, but there are other situations that we can only do so much about.

Taylor: My drunk dad had this prayer on his dresser for years, but I never thought it would be helpful for me.

Jillian: It can be very empowering. Basically for the situations we cannot do anything about, it can be helpful to utilize this mindset of letting go. This means that instead of getting emotionally entrenched in circumstances we may have no control over, we let them be.

One way to do this is to imagine yourself turning an unmanageable situation over to someone or something else to take care of it. As an example, younger children may have difficulty imagining this, so therapists often invite them to hand over their worries and fears. Some therapists even suggest that they will store the child's fears in a box in their office. The concept is that by releasing them from our sole possession, we're acknowledging there is only so much we can do about some things. At this point, we are inviting the help of someone or something else, be it a higher power, a force of nature, a friend, or a therapist.

Min: This is an interesting concept for the topic of control. It does seem like it offers you a choice to be safe even when you have no certainty about what will be occurring. All of this kind of reminds me of what my grandfather used to tell my father about his business. It goes something like this: "You have no control over anything or anybody. Know this, believe this, and accept this."

The letting go piece seems very comforting and freeing to me – I like it.

Jillian: Min, thank you for sharing your grandfather's wise words. They resonate with another element of finding healthy control that I would like to introduce to all of you.

I would like to introduce a strategy you can use to help you communicate your needs and desires more effectively to other people. It is called assertive communication. **Assertive communication exhibits healthy control.** It is used not only as a tool in therapy to assist with effective communication, but also used as a model in parenting classes, utilized in mediation training, and taught as a fundamental skill in business management courses.

I have adapted a particular model form Edmund Bourne's *Anxiety and Phobia Workbook*. This has been used by my colleagues with many of their clients The basic idea here is by learning to communicate to others in a clear and non-offensive way, you can be an active agent of change in your life, and you can take more control over the situations you can change. Listen and relax, even close your eyes if you would like, while I read this adaptation to all of you.

There is a big difference between communicating needs and feelings assertively and aggressively. When we communicate aggressively, our intention is either to win, to vent, or to hurt someone. When communicating assertively, our goal is to solve a problem or strengthen a relationship. It is an opportunity for both people to gain something.

Steps to Communicate Assertively
Make a plan.

It is Okay to tell someone you need time to think before responding to a situation. You may also need time to calm down or vent your feelings to someone else first. You may want to write them down ahead of time to organize your thoughts. Figure out ahead of time what you want to say and how and when to say it.

Tell the truth.

Speak form your heart and tell what's true for that moment. Try to be kind and unhurtful.

Try following the guidelines of using "Direct I Statements."

I see…(What have you observed or noticed)

I think…(How you see it)

I feel…

I need…(What you would like the person to do instead) Listen to the response.

It is important to stay centered and respectful and to focus on relaxing and breathing. If the other person is disrespectful, you can return to the format and tell them how their behaviors are making you feel right now. "When you yell at me like this, I feel scared and upset..." If things don't calm down, you can always say you are not willing to continue and leave.

Work on solutions. Offer a solution, and try to be willing to compromise.

I know this can sound very overwhelming and complicated, but it really isn't. Let's try to practice this, and then it may become clearer. I wonder is there anyone that has a certain situation they want to practice being assertive with?

Taylor: I definitely do!

Jillian: Okay, Taylor, why don't you explain to us the situation you would like to be more assertive with.

Taylor: The situation I want to use has to do with my boyfriend. He gets really upset when I spend time with people other than him. He yells and screams, and then he ends up walking off or driving away, and then I get furious. It is ridiculous!

Jillian: So if you were to follow the assertive communication model, what could you do?

Taylor: Tell him what I see?

Jillian: Yes. What would that sound like?

Taylor: I think like this. When I go out with my friends, you get really angry at me and blow up.

Jillian: Good and what do you think?

Taylor: I think this happens because you care about me and you get worried that if I'm with other people, they'll be a bad influence on me or take me away from you.

Jillian: Great, Taylor. Now, the *I feel…*

Taylor: I get really upset when this happens because I care about you a lot, but I miss my friends. What if we plan out a schedule where I'm with them on certain days and you on others?

Jillian: That was well done, Taylor.

Taylor: Thanks – but I've never had a conversation like that in my life.

Stephanie: As I listened, it really seemed the way you were talking, Taylor, could really help to solve this issue between you and your boyfriend.

Taylor: God, that would be nice!

Jillian: I wonder what other thoughts there are after observing this demonstration of assertive communication.

Min: I feel very empowered by this. I was never taught anything like this growing up because in my family an assertive woman many times is labeled as disrespectful. This, though, is a very respectful way to be assertive. I really cannot wait to have an opportunity to experiment with it.

Jillian: How wonderful for you to realize that there is a voice in you begging to speak. I hope you find this effective in giving yourself more freedom to be who you really are.
      Carly, do you have anything you would like to add or share?

Carly: I think it is a great thought if you know what you need or want to communicate. My life feels so busy and fast most of the time, I have no idea what is happening for me.

Jillian: Carly, that is very honest of you. As you continue on in your journey of recovery it will become easier for you to channel more of your focus and energy inward on yourself. Then I imagine you will be able to offer yourself the gift of assertive communication.

Carly: Hopefully someday.

Jillian: You have all done quite a bit of work here again this evening. The topic of control is very complex in the role it can play in life with an eating disorder. Hopefully, each of you may be developing a better understanding of why this is such a central issue and also observe how control relates to your individual life circumstances and how it may impact your behaviors. As you all leave here tonight, I would like everyone to take the kindness and support you received here, from each other, and offer some towards yourself. Recovery from and eating disorder is hard work. Please enjoy this evening's *Words of Hope*.

> Some of us are faced with more challenge than we know what to do with, and we lose our way. If we can hold on long enough to embrace a hand that can help lead us to safety, then it is we who, in turn, become the light.

Before we end, just a reminder that next time we meet, our usual group format will be slightly different because we will be having a special guest speaker sharing with us her story of recovery. We will reserve the first half hour for our group, and then we will welcome our guest.

Have a nice week.

Week Six

One Woman's Recovery

Throughout my years of nursing experience, it has been very clear that listening to stories of another person's recovery can truly aide in the recovery experience for many.

By listening and sharing personal stories, there is an honesty and authenticity that exists. Oftentimes, this helps diminish the sense of isolation that is present for many who have an eating disorder. It is also an effective approach for challenging discussions to occur. For example, I have often seen the difficult and threatening topic of **hospitalization** (often necessary to break the destructive cycle of an eating disorder and provide an opportunity for recovery) effectively discussed in this type of sharing.

In the group setting, many times a guest speaker who has struggled through recovery provides a road map to health for others. I believe that hearing the struggles and triumphs of others does promote a true sense of hope.

Managing One Woman's Recovery

It appears some young women may feel threatened by listening to the reality of another person's experience. I make it known in the groups I facilitate, that if an issue or topic is discussed and becomes disturbing to an individual, it is important to examine this further with myself or their individual therapist. I do believe even in this type of circumstance, individuals can still receive incite that over time offers them strength throughout their recovery process.

My belief in the effectiveness of group therapy for the treatment of eating disorders is supported by the capacity many young women demonstrate when they come together and listen to the stories of others, while identifying with their own struggles. For many this is a critical piece in an effective journey through recovery.

Have you ever listened to another women's story of recovery? I think it is important to understand that observing another speak about their own eating disorder struggles can bring about different changes within you at different phases of your own recovery. Allow yourself the understanding that at one time listening to another's story may be too triggering, yet a few weeks later it may be just the support you are looking for. As this Week evolves, notice what is happening within yourself. Is the voice of your eating disorder chatting louder to you? Or are you being filled with hope and some excitement at the possibility of change?

As you were talking, I felt like you could be telling
my story. So much of what you said reminds me of me.

– Taylor

Jillian: Welcome back to all of you. Have you noticed it is light out tonight as we meet? The season change is becoming more evident.

Carly: I love how the sun comes through these windows and warms all of us with its light. The room was bright, but now it seems brilliant. It feels nice being here.

Jillian: That is a very inspirational statement, Carly, and it is nice to recognize that it feels good to you when you are here.
As we begin I would like to remind all of you this is Week

Six and as I mentioned last week much of our group time this evening will be shared with our special guest speaker.

Anika: Can you tell us a little about her?

Jillian: Her name is Elisabeth Perkins. She has been a friend and colleague of mine for many years. She is a parent, school teacher, and is actively involved in many efforts to raise community awareness and promote education on eating disorders. She has been kind enough to join us this evening and share with us her story of recovery from Anorexia.

Taylor fidgets, pulling her skirt down to cover her legs.

Taylor: I don't mean to interrupt, but can I sit on the floor with a pillow – these stupid chairs just don't agree with me and my body. Ugh!

Jillian: Sure, Taylor. I kept our circle of chairs and just added one extra for our guest. For all of you, do whatever you need to be comfortable.

Is this more comfortable for you, Taylor?

Taylor: For now. I'm just having some insecure fat feelings today.

Jillian: Taylor, would you like to tell us more about that.

Taylor: It's hard for me sometimes. I mean, I know you all now and am used to you, but at our first few groups I felt very uncomfortable and gross about my body when we met. I guess having somebody I don't know who is or was Anorexic makes me feel insecure or threatened somehow. Damn – I am psycho!

Jillian: I can assure you that you are not psycho, Taylor. You just demonstrated great awareness of yourself. Good for you! In fact I am so glad you introduced this point to the group. I wonder if you all have thought about the competitive thoughts and feelings that may drive your eating disorders at times.

Many young women find being around others with eating disorders can be triggering. It's almost as if you can become territorial about your coping mechanism of food, weight, body image, etc. I invited this particular guest because I believe you'll feel very comfortable with Elisabeth. She will present her story, without all the details that maybe triggering and she understands on a personal level how uncomfortable listening to another's story can be. Then you all will have an opportunity to ask her questions. If anyone feels uncomfortable during this group, at any time, it is important to let me know.

Taylor, I am glad you allowed yourself the opportunity to discuss the anxiety you are experiencing being here tonight. Talk with me if there is anything else you may need.

Taylor: Thanks. Sorry to be so high maintenance.

Jillian: Needs are not high maintenance.

Min: I hope this doesn't sound disrespectful, but if being around others with eating disorder issues can be triggering, why would you want a speaker to come into our group?

Jillian: What a wonderful question.

In my years of working with young women with eating disorders, I have found it is one thing to hear theories about recovery and another to listen to a person's actual story. By being in this group, you may be well aware that telling stories is a useful and meaningful tool, especially when someone is seeking guidance and inspiration. Within this journey of recovery, oftentimes it can feel as though you are losing your way and there is no guide book to direct you back home. I am hoping by presenting you with Elisabeth's story of recovery, you may be able to use her experiences to help you find your way.

Min: That makes sense.

Jillian: Are there any other thoughts or comments?

Our guest is waiting down the hall in the waiting area and now I think it would be a good time to invite her into our group for this evening. If it is okay, I am just going to open the white door of this room and welcome her in.

Jillian opens the door and invites the speaker to join the group.
Please welcome Elisabeth Perkins.

Elisabeth: Hello everyone. What a beautiful space you all meet in.

I want to thank you for giving me this opportunity. I am honored to be in the company of such strong and courageous women. And although I know very little about you, I do know you are here because you have the desire to recover. You have the openness of heart and mind to discover new and healthier ways to live your lives, and for that you are to be highly commended.

Before I begin, would you all mind, at the very least, introducing yourselves? After we go around the circle, I promise to get started, and then you'll have plenty of time at the end to ask me questions.

Carly: I'll start. Hi. I'm Carly!

Min: My name is Min. Thank you for being here.

Anika: I am Anika.

Stephanie: Welcome to our group. My name is Stephanie.

Taylor: I'm Taylor.

Elisabeth: It is a pleasure to meet all of you.

If it feels okay to everyone, I would like to begin.

I think I will start at the beginning. For me, my eating disorder began earlier than it does for most people. I was only nine years old. And when I think back about how it all got started, it's now clear to me it wasn't just one thing that was responsible for causing it. The seeds were probably there for many years, if not from birth, but it required the right soil and environment to really take hold. I was always a people pleaser and always very conscious of making certain everyone around me was happy. I hated conflict, tension, or arguments of any kind, and I was going to make sure I was never the one responsible for causing them. However, when there was a conflict, even when it had nothing to do with me, I did feel responsible. So I went along in my very young life, acutely aware of the way my family responded to me and to each other. I was always trying to stay one step ahead of them to prevent any oncoming problems. I avoided anger at all costs – mine and theirs. On the

Week Six: One Woman's Recovery

outside, everything was fine, but on the inside, I was an anxious mess. I worried about everything and needed everything around me to be perfect...especially me. I hid my frustration, anger, anxiety, and sadness so well that after enough time had elapsed, even I had no idea what I was really feeling.

In looking back, this need for perfection began even earlier. At age four, I remember taking dance and spending hour upon hour practicing the steps in my room until I could get them right. And yet they never seemed good enough. In elementary school, I had to make sure the teachers all loved me, and I could get nothing below an A. My clothes and hair had to be perfect. I couldn't tolerate the idea of disappointing anyone at any time. I think you're probably getting the picture.

Nine was a pivotal age for me. Although my looks had been important, they became more of an obsession. People always told me I was cute and I should have been a model, even at age nine, and I enjoyed the attention. I began to believe it was a person's looks that really mattered in life, and this was soon to be reinforced through my peers, television, and magazines. I compared myself to everyone, and I never felt like I measured up.

Inside, I felt I was different from everyone. They never seemed to have the worries I did, or didn't appear to, and I felt like an outsider. And so, these were the seeds...

At age nine, two events then occurred in my life that changed the way I experienced my world and furthered the process of my downward spiral. Both of my mother's parents were diagnosed with Cancer within a couple of months of each other, and she needed to care for them. My mother and I had been extremely close, and the idea of her going away for days at a time to take care of them seemed intolerable. I missed her terribly. The fact that I had no control over the health of my grandparents, or the amount of time my mother needed to be away, only compounded my anxiety.

During this time, my family tried to retain as much of a sense of normalcy as possible. My brother and I went to school and participated in our after school extracurricular activities, but my need for control and perfection only tightened its strangling grip. I was athletic, and I enjoyed seeing the results of my physical hard work. What I didn't enjoy was the fact that my body built muscle very easily and my legs felt like those of a sumo wrestler. I was extremely self-conscious about the size I perceived them to be.

The development of my eating disorder behaviors began in the third grade. I remember it being field day at school, but I couldn't go because I was at home with the stomach flu. I was in bed all day, unable to eat. I remember I watched TV all day and saw countless commercials about losing weight. They gave the message, "Lose weight and you'll be happy." So I began figuring out how many calories I had for the day, which wasn't many because I was sick. I then wrote them down on a tissue box near my bed. This had become my new obsession.

Over the next few months, my life continued to change dramatically. I have a memory of being at the movies and deciding to buy Raisinets instead of other candy because they were "less caloric" and were fruit. Restricting calories became all I would think about. I was now mirror obsessed, and although my world depended on how I looked, it was never good enough. I compared myself to everyone and matched up to no one. My Anorexia spun out of control, and I grew sicker and sicker. I lived in my own obsessed and lonely world. And yet I lied, pushed away, and abused those whom I loved in order to protect the "safe" world I had created. I was unhappy and depressed. I hated myself and took my hatred out on food and myself. If I couldn't punch myself or hit my head, I would angrily rip the food that was prepared for me into little pieces. When I was upset, I would take it out on my looks. At my lowest point, I would stay in bed all day and only allow myself one thing to eat.

When I was thirteen, I was hospitalized for the first time at Boston Children's Hospital. I was placed on the Psychiatric Unit, and from the moment I was admitted there, my every move was monitored. I was terrified by the prospect of having to give up any of my self-destructive behaviors and frightened that I could not be with my family. I was no longer in control. If I refused to eat, I was given a supplemental drink. If my refusal lasted too long, they would threaten me with a feeding tube. Here I was, in as extreme a setting as I could possibly be, and I still thought everyone was overreacting in their concern.

Unfortunately, my length of stay there was dictated by what the insurance company viewed as medically, not psychologically, necessary. Therefore, as soon as my weight had gone up enough to meet their medical criteria, I was discharged home.

Shortly after arriving home, I returned to my unhealthy behaviors full throttle. The main difference, however, was it didn't seem to feel quite as beneficial as it did before. I think while I was hospitalized the healthier part of me, which was in there somewhere, had had a chance to grow a little stronger. Unfortunately though, it wasn't strong enough to overpower the eating disorder voice – or the behaviors that followed.

At age sixteen, I returned to Boston Children's Hospital more depleted, physically and emotionally, than I ever had been. This time, I was sufficiently scared, and I felt incapable of making any of the behaviors stop, even though I knew I would have to in order to survive. I remember one of the nurses telling me that if I continued along this path much longer, I would either die or ruin my chances to ever have children. She told me this was the only body I would ever have. I wanted to have children one day, and this conversation seemed to permeate my eating disorder fog and increase my desire to get better.

I wasn't getting better in this setting though, and in the meantime, my individual therapist, along with my parents, agreed it was a good idea to have me transferred to another hospital that was more specialized in eating disorders. This one was in Vermont. The insurance company refused to pay for it and wanted to send me home. I have vague memories of my father having to go in front of a judge in order to appeal this decision. I realized, at this point, that if I returned home for any period of time, I might not survive. The fight within me was weakening. I felt alone, lost, and helpless.

I was admitted to a substance abuse unit at the hospital in

Vermont, shortly thereafter. This was the case because there were no beds available on the eating disorder unit. I was younger than most of the people there, and no one else had an eating disorder. As I listened to them talk about their addictions and their recovery, I continued to feel alone and lost. This was supposed to be the place where I was going to get the help I needed.

Finally, during one of the therapy groups, I was listening to someone reading the Twelve Steps, and something took hold. I found great comfort in the idea of surrendering my eating disorder over to a "Higher Power" of some kind. I had been raised Catholic, yet I hadn't been very religious, but somehow it was the spiritual fabric of the twelve step program that was now providing me with new strength and courage. I would sit at meals with the other patients and hear them talking about prayer and "acting as if." They advised me to do what they had been told: to act as if you believed in prayer, in getting healthy, and in the spiritual part of the program, even if you didn't. They said it would help me get better. So I prayed and I read affirmations. I prayed and read more affirmations. I wrote down all the many things people had told me, on whatever paper I could find, that I thought might help me to recover. I posted them all over my room, and I carried them with me.

Within this setting, my recovery finally began to take hold. The healthy voice grew stronger, along with my body, now strong enough to begin to stand up to the unhealthy voice. I remember someone had told me not to let the eating disorder voice have the last word in our arguments and to turn my anger toward what was making me unhealthy instead of myself. I continued with my obsessions and my rituals, but with much less intensity.

I eventually returned home, transferring all my affirmations from the walls in the hospital to the walls of my bedroom. And so, I clung to my therapy sessions and all the support I could muster. I fought for my life, one meal at a time, with the conviction that if I returned to my destructive ways, there would be no coming back.

My full recovery was challenging, but perhaps what was even harder to accept was the realization that I had given up several good years of my life to my eating disorder. It took me a long time to forgive myself for this. However, when I finally did forgive myself, I realized my eating disorder had been instrumental in helping me to discover ways to live a healthy and peaceful life. This challenge has also provided me with the passion and desire to help others.

I want to thank everyone for listening to my story of recovery and for being here. If you all feel comfortable I would like to take this time to discuss what it may have been like for you to listen to me talk about my struggles and recovery.

Taylor: When you began, I felt really uncomfortable, fat, and threatened. Then as you were talking, I felt like you could be telling my story. So much of what you said reminds me of me.

I have a question: What was it like for you with your parents when you got home from the hospital?

Elisabeth: Up until I came out of the last hospitalization I don't think my parents understood and knew what to do for me. But, by that point, from numerous family meetings and therapy sessions, they were really good at knowing the best ways to support me. For the longest time, I ate all of my meals with some kind of meal support. Someone was always there to remind me in a gentle way what my goals were, to distract me while I ate, or to go for a walk or play a game after I ate. This would help me take my mind off of how full or uncomfortable I felt.

Taylor: But didn't it feel like they were mothering you and trying to control you?

Elisabeth: At the time no, because by then I wanted to fight my eating disorder. I tried to use my family like I used the nurses at Brattleboro – for strength, distraction, and support. Yet prior to this when I wasn't ready to recover, yes, any involvement my parents had with my food created much more difficultly for me.

Stephanie: You are so honest in your speaking. I also really identified with your story.

I was wondering if you could talk a little about whether or not they put you on any kind of medication, and if they did, was it helpful?

Elisabeth: Medication was a big part of my recovery. It helped quiet some of the anxiety and despair. I was started on it when I was eleven, but it wasn't really until I was sixteen that they finally had me on the right combinations of medication. At that point, I was able to get some of the obsessions and compulsions under control.

Stephanie: Wow, that is a long time to get the right combination.

Elisabeth: Yes it was, but it fits the flux and change that recovery involves. What I am trying to say is, I had to get to the point where I was really ready to recover, then things like medication and coping skills became truly effective.

Stephanie: Thanks for explaining that, it helps.

Elisabeth: I'm so glad. Are there any other questions?

Carly: I do. I feel like I'm saying the same things as everyone else, but we all have so many parallels.

You don't look like someone that went through all of that. What do you think the hardest part of recovery was?

Elisabeth: Probably making the commitment to get better and then sticking to it. Upon leaving the hospital, I actually wrote out and signed a contract with myself that said no matter how tough things got, I would not go back to old behaviors.

Taylor: And did you?

Elisabeth: On occasion, I would slip back, but I would quickly pull myself up again. I firmly believed if I let myself slip too much for too long, I wouldn't have the strength to get myself back out again. In the past, with each setback I had, I became sicker and weaker, and the road out seemed that much more treacherous and impossible to navigate. I didn't know if I would make it again. Also the eating disorder just wasn't satisfying me or comforting me like it used to. I was getting tired of it.

Yet, another really difficult part of the commitment that existed for me was I was so fearful of giving up my identity as someone with an eating disorder. I didn't know who I was without it. I was afraid people wouldn't like me if they really got to know the "true" me.

Taylor: I know what you mean. I feel like my eating disorder makes me important in some weird ways. Without it, I would be nothing.

Elisabeth: Yes, I understand that very well. The one thing that I discovered is the eating disorder did cover parts of me up for years and this was comforting then. But eventually, as I went through different parts of my recovery and learned more about myself, I craved more of the "real" me – the part hidden by the eating disorder. One of the most effective ways for me to work through this was with the affirmations I collected, that I spoke about earlier.

Carly: Would you please share some of those with us?

Elisabeth: I would feel honored. I actually brought a list of my favorites that I found most helpful. I will just read them to you all. See how they sit in you as you hear them.

I'm not my body, I'm my personality

Let my body decide what I want

Accept my body and looks the way they are now

A non-anorexic life = living life, not wasting life

Take chances, the fear will pay off

I'm hungry, so I eat despite the crazy thoughts

Change is never comfortable

Say my feelings

Being healthy is beautiful

Take care of myself

Take a break and let loose

When I feel like giving in to the Anorexia, I think of all
the good times and fun I could have if I was well

Don't wait!

It's hard, it's scary, but hold on for the next day, the
next moment, the next meal

The Anorexic me is a lie and tortuous self

I need to build up my self-esteem, not by losing
weight, but by figuring out who I really am

Help me to love and respect me

What does everyone think?

Carly: I love them. I felt like they spoke directly to me.

Stephanie: I agree, they sound and feel so empowering.

Anika: For me, I can relate to a few of them. Although I feel
strange trying to think of myself in such positive ways, listening to these statements allows me to think that is possible to
figure out who I really am and what I truly want.

Taylor: I think they are cool. But for me, they don't fit. They are
too nice for me. Maybe someday though, I won't be so imbalanced and I can see the world and myself in a better light.

Elisabeth: I am so glad you all received something from the affirmations.

Are there other thoughts?

Min: Yes, I do. First of all, thank you for being so candid. It is
very helpful.

I was wondering, what were the most important things you
learned?

Elisabeth: To begin with, I learned that I had all of these im-

Week Six: One Woman's Recovery   151

portant feelings inside and how to express them. I learned how to be alone and to actually enjoy it. I learned the art of nurturing and taking care of myself. I learned how to relax and that coping skills really work when you decide to use them. I also discovered it was important to figure out the purpose my eating disorder played in my life, but I didn't necessarily need to know exactly what caused my eating disorder in order to recover. I just needed to work on trusting the process. One of the best lessons was realizing that all the new ways of thinking and coping that I developed would not only help in my recovery, but would also allow me to live a healthier and happier life, long after the ties to my eating disorder were severed.

Anika: Elisabeth, I have a question. Something I haven't fully understood. It sounds like the hospitalizations played a really big role in your recovery. Why do you think they were so important?

Elisabeth: I believe the structure of the hospital gave me a chance to grow a healthier part of me I didn't know I had. Each time I was admitted, the healthier part had a chance to get a little stronger, even though it wasn't immediately apparent. They also helped my body to get nourished and become physically stronger. Without my physical strength and adequate number of calories, I wouldn't have been able to see the pathway to recovery. My brain wasn't working well enough. Each time I was hospitalized, all of my control around food was taken away. As excruciating as this was, it allowed me some rest even though I rebelled against this, there were parts of me that welcomed it. I hope that answers your question.

Anika: Yes, it does. Thank you.

Carly: I have something else I would like to ask. I hope this doesn't sound too intrusive, but could you tell us a little about your life now?
Are you ever tempted to slip back?
Do you struggle with your body image?

Elisabeth: You aren't being intrusive at all. I'm really glad you asked that. I'm now twenty-eight and very happily married. I have a little girl who is eighteen months old, and she is the joy of my life. I work part-time as an early childhood teacher, and when I can get away, I occasionally lecture on eating disorders. I am still very much of a perfectionist at heart, and a worrier, but I have learned how to let go of things. I have discovered much healthier ways to cope with my feelings. As far as my body image goes, I have come to accept the woman I am, with all its flaws and imperfections. I do the best I can with what I have to work with, but my priority is more about being the person I want to be. I am proud of the fact that my body has the amazing capacity to give and to sustain life.

Carly: That's so amazing and hopeful. Thank you!

Elisabeth: You are welcome.

I want you all to realize, no two recoveries look the same. What I mean is, each person's recovery will unfold differently. Remember, this is your unique experience and your life. Let it become what you want it to be.

Stephanie: I think that is so true.

I'm sorry, I am back tracking, but you mentioned that several factors contributed to your eating disorder, however, in looking back now, is there any one thing you think could really have prevented all of your suffering or at least made it easier?

Elisabeth: I mentioned a little about this, but I didn't go into it very deeply. I apologize.

I mentioned that my family was Catholic, and although I maintained some of the religious practices and beliefs, I still felt a huge void in my life. Something was missing and I couldn't quite figure out what it was. As I got older, I realized that although there was a religious presence, there was no spiritual presence in my life. I had no idea what my purpose in life was or how I fit in with the greater scheme of things. I had no belief in myself and no awareness of the interconnectedness of life.

Taylor: You completely lost me. Can you explain more about that spiritual part that was missing and how you were able to figure it out?

Elisabeth: Sure. I realize these are difficult concepts to grasp, and they probably sound a little strange. I will try to be a bit clearer.

I was never aware that inside of me I had an inner spirit, an inner self that needed to be paid attention to and nourished. No one ever told me this. I was never aware of there being a connection between my mind, body, and spirit. But in my last hospitalization, I was given the challenge of looking ahead to my future. I was asked to explore "Where would I like to see myself five years from now?", "Ten years from now?" I really think shifting my thoughts this way allowed me some space that helped me realize there was a deeper part of myself.

It wasn't really until I was an adult and I was taking a yoga class that I experienced the true connection. I began doing yoga when I became pregnant with my daughter. Finally, I felt this void in myself filled. The connection I felt between my mind, my body, and my breath helped me discover my place in this world.

I have continued to practice yoga and meditation and I realize that by having a spiritual perspective in my life, I am able to stay grounded, regardless of what is going on. It provides a sense of inner calm and peace that in turn allows me to remain in touch with who I truly am and what I may need.

Taylor, I hope that is a better explanation for you.

Taylor: Yes, thanks. It is more clear, but very deep.

Elisabeth: That's true it is.

I see it is getting very late and I don't want to take up too much more of your time together. If there are no more questions or thoughts I will let Jillian continue with your group.

Jillian: Thank you, Elisabeth. I appreciate you being a part of our group this evening. Your story is truly inspiring.

I was wondering if it would be Okay with all you girls if

Elisabeth ended the group with us this evening by listening to the Words of Hope. What does everyone think?

Carly: I think that would be great! Thank you again, Elisabeth.

Min: Yes, it would feel awkward for you to leave now. Thank you for being so real – it is inspiring.

Elisabeth: It has been an honor. Now what are these words of hope?

Jillian: *Words of Hope* are inspirational thoughts that I read to the girls, at the end of each group, to close our time together and hopefully send some empowering thoughts with all of us, as we transition into the moments and week that follow.

Elisabeth: That sounds beautiful. I would love to be a part of this closing ritual.

Jillian: I wonder this evening if we could all join hands as I read. If you are comfortable enough to do so, please join hands with the person next to you. If not it is fine to just listen.

When we listen to the stories of others, both struggles and triumphs, we allow parts of ourselves to be challenged and nurtured. May the stories that you share here, evolve into the unique biographies that you all crave. Be the author and create the masterpiece that you desire.

Thank you all for sharing this special group with me. I look forward to our next time together next week.

Carly: May I walk out with you, Elisabeth?

Elisabeth: That would be fine. I would love to walk into the next moment with all of you if you wish.

Week Seven

Hungers

While working with young women recovering from eating disorders, it is apparent that there are hungers or deficiencies in their life, a piece that is missing. They often appear to use their eating disorder to satisfy this void by being filled up or trying to escape from it.

Some of these girls may come from emotional neglect, abuse, or a home where a parental figure is missing. Many of these young women who have Anorexia, Bulimia, or Binge-eating disorder feel separate from the world around them. This then creates or adds to their sense of isolation and low self-esteem.

I recognize that many of these young women do not know how to fill this void. **They experience what I recognize as a hunger for connection – a connection to meaning, life, people, interests, and spirituality.**

Managing Hungers

It appears with proper support, from a therapeutic team approach (which includes a Physician, Psychiatrist, Therapist, and a Nutritionist), it is possible for many of these young women to satisfy their hungers in healthy ways. This is a life skill that not only benefits their recovery but also living a healthy, fulfilling life beyond the eating disorder.

Dealing with these hungers involves creating opportunities for these young women to get to know themselves on a deeper level, while nurturing themselves, and finding what has meaning for them. When they are able to find their meaning in life, they discover more purpose and opportunity. They are also able to rely on themselves more confidently to fulfill their own expectations.

What do you truly hunger for? For you, this question may be simple to answer, or you may not even be able to connect with the thought that you are craving connections. As you continue to receive support from members of your therapeutic team, it will become clear that you are worthy of receiving what you most deeply need from yourself and others. I encourage you to witness the girls in the group explore this issue. See if their experiences assist you with learning about your own personal connections and what may be lacking for you.

The empty feeling you guys describe sounds just like what I have felt so much of my life. Maybe it has something to do with my father traveling and not being around all the time.

– Min

Jillian: Welcome. It is hard to believe it is week seven of our group.

How is everyone doing?

Taylor: I'm sorry, but I hope nobody minds if I take off my shoes. These damn high heel shoes have been killing my feet all day.

Taylor slips off her leopard print high heel shoes and places them under her chair.

The price I pay to stay attractive.

Jillian: It is fine, Taylor, make yourself as comfortable as you can.

Min: Excuse me, Jillian, but I couldn't help noticing the beautiful Forsythia bouquet on the bookshelf. Are they real?

Jillian: Yes they are. I am glad you noticed them.

Today when I was walking my dog I collected some. The brightness of the flower captured my eye. It was as if, out of the dark gray days of winter something vibrant appeared. I immediately thought of this group. You all have this vibrant part of yourself waiting to come out. I have seen glimpses of this in each and every one of you. Allow yourselves to witness and be embraced by the bright energy of this flower as we begin our group this evening.

Who would like to start by telling us how things have been going.

Taylor: I would like to begin. By the way the flowers are really pretty. Too bad my life can't be.

What a roller coaster this week has been! Get this, I found out my boyfriend was cheating on me, and so we broke up, but then last night he called me and told me he couldn't live without me. He said he realizes he was such a jerk, and he's sorry for hurting me. He said he had been drinking with friends and things just got out of hand. We're Okay now. Actually, we're coming up on our three month anniversary, and he wants to take me out to a fancy restaurant. That makes me really nervous. I'm not a big fan of restaurants – obviously!

Stephanie: Can I ask you something, Taylor?

Taylor: Sure.

Stephanie: Isn't this the second time you've caught him cheating on you?

Taylor: Yeah, but he promises that she meant nothing to him, and he knows he was a jerk.

Min: Taylor, I think you could do so much better.

Taylor: Not really. I have so many hang-ups. I have no talents. I'm fat. I don't even know why he wants to be with me in the first place.

Jillian: Taylor, it sounds very difficult what you have had to deal with. It also sounds very painful to have such negative self talk.

Taylor: It sucks – but I'm used to putting myself down. All my life whenever anything goes wrong, I think if I were different, better, more attractive, then things may not be so crappy. I'm used to feeling lousy about myself. I guess it's all I know.

Anika: Wow, you and I sure are lacking in self-confidence! It's funny how it's so easy to see each other's strengths and be able to realize what would be best for each other, but it's so hard to see it in ourselves.

Taylor, you are kind, witty, beautiful, and filled with spirit – and your boyfriend doesn't realize what he's got. We really don't need men as much as we think we do. In fact, they only complicate matters, and they can be such jerks. I'm beginning to realize I have to live my life for myself and no one else – not my family and not a man.

In fact, I have been doing a lot of thinking this week, and I have had some moments when I've felt really strong. I'm actually thinking about getting a better paying job and moving into my own apartment and finding a roommate. That's in a stronger moment. In a weaker one, I start wondering what I was thinking and who I'm kidding. "You can't live on your own without your family. You're irresponsible and careless, and you'd never be able to pull this off." Then the fears and what ifs start to bombard me. What if I got lonely, and what if I'm just fooling myself into thinking I'm ready to handle independence? Is this self-doubt related to my parents and my upbringing? I feel like I hold myself back – no one else does. I have no belief in myself, but I'm really good at helping others know what to do. My parents criticize everything I do, and they always have. They have no faith in me.

Taylor: It's nice to know you understand.

Anika: I totally do.

Jillian: Wow, you girls have done a great job describing important observations of yourselves related to self-esteem.

Anika: Would you explain a bit about how our self-esteem becomes no self-esteem.

Jillian: Of course.

Our self-esteem begins developing from the time that we are very young. **It is that part of us from which we draw our strength and the belief that we are capable, worthwhile beings.** If the people who are significant to us have little faith in us or our abilities, it becomes difficult to have it in ourselves. Many girls with eating disorders totally underestimate themselves and their self-worth.

Carly: So, do you think it's just families that are responsible for this, because my family was always so supportive – at least as far as I can remember.

Jillian: Actually, many things can undermine the development of self-esteem, of development in general, for that matter.

If someone grows up in a setting of instability and chaos, where one's needs are rarely recognized or met, growth – in terms of healthy emotional development – can be interrupted. If our caregivers are unable to validate the importance of our thoughts, feelings, and needs, it becomes difficult for us to internalize our own sense of worth and importance. Also, as children, if our role models themselves are struggling with their own self-esteem we can learn to mirror similar struggles.

Taylor: Tell me about it.

Jillian: It sounds like you can relate to what I am saying, Taylor.

Also, unhealthy relationships with our peers or even a partner may undermine the development and sustenance of self-esteem. If we surround ourselves with people who are continually critical and ostracizing, we can begin internalizing extreme self-doubt.

Min: Is it just relationships that really alter our esteem?

Jillian: No, in fact emotional challenges like chronic anxiety and depression can also color the way we see the world and ourselves in it. When we live in perpetual fear or hopelessness, we begin to lose faith in our own abilities and of those around us.

Moreover, there is the impact that culture can have on self-esteem. For example, if women are repeatedly given a cultural message they are not as worthy as men, or that it is their looks and not their ideas and beliefs that contribute to success, this can undermine personal worth and achievement.

Carly: I'm really beginning to understand all of this in a new way. It seems like the setting has got be right for an eating disorder to take hold or develop in someone, almost like the fertile soil in Elisabeth's story.

Jillian: Yes, certain characteristics or external influences seem to put a person at higher risk for developing an eating disorder. Low self-esteem can create an atmosphere for self criticism to grow wildly, and it can also make you feel personally responsible for anything that goes wrong in your life.

Carly: Is there any way to build up self-esteem?

Jillian: Yes. The thing about self-esteem is it can definitely get trodden upon – and the effects can be truly damaging. However, it's one of those things like our hearts – in time and in the right setting, we can mend. Many of the skills we have been learning here together each week can help you strengthen your belief in who you are.

In fact, I will read you a list of some additional ideas I have collected over the years. I like to call these ideas *Suggestions for Building Self-Esteem.*

Listen to your inner thoughts and feelings

Pay attention to your needs and try to make plans to accommodate them

Nurture yourself on a daily basis

Develop the kind of support that will give you feelings of confidence, self-respect, and acceptance

Try not to forget about the importance of reminding others about your need for boundaries and limits

Include in your schedule, time to take care of your physical well being. This might include exercising moderately, taking time to plan for meals and shop for food, or making necessary doctor's appointments

Leave time for emotional self-expression, positive self-talk, and affirmations

Make it a point to remember your personal accomplishments

Take challenges you think will lead to your feeling better about yourself

Do what you can, as best you can, for this day

And try to remember: all of this is an ongoing process, so you don't have to do it all perfectly

That is what being kind to yourself can be.
What does everyone think?

Carly: It sounds so nice.

Min: I could really feel the love and respect that is involved with these suggestions.

Stephanie: It is very inviting to think of living like that, but part of me sees it as being selfish.

Taylor: When I was listening to you, I felt all weird inside imaging being so nice to myself.

Anika: For me, it's a little of what everyone has said.

Jillian: I am glad reading this to all of you has stimulated your thinking related to your individual self-esteems. Remember, the process of recovery involves many factors, including this. So, being patient and gentle with yourselves as you work through your journey is a wonderful start for rebuilding self-esteem.

Stephanie, I don't want to put you on the spot, but you look like you want to say something.

Stephanie: I do. It might be related to this or not, but I have been waiting for Tuesday to come so I could talk about what's been going on.

Jillian: Go ahead.

Stephanie: I've been doing really well for several weeks now, which for me is quite amazing. Even the pull to restrict is beginning to loosen its grip. But this terrifies me. I should be happy, but I'm not. I feel like I'm beginning to grieve for a friend that's leaving soon. It's been such a part of my life for so long, and in thinking back, it has been one way, one of the only ways, that I have gotten any attention. Well, maybe that's an exaggeration – enough attention. Not that I did this deliberately, but it made people pay attention.

Jillian: Although I feel excited for you that you are noticing a shift in the role your eating disorder has in your life, I also understand your concern.

In the groups I have facilitated, many young women have often expressed a feeling of being passed over in life or forgotten about. This phenomenon often occurs because of their low self-esteem and because they feel unworthy of recognition. For them, their eating disorder can call forth an opportunity to be seen and cared for, not to suggest that this is a deliberate act, but more of a secondary gain they soon learn to depend on.

Stephanie: Exactly, I mean I always felt like I was invisible, even in school. I was quiet. I remember thinking that if I didn't attract any attention from my teachers I was doing them a favor, because they always seemed so stressed. I guess in some ways I did the same thing at home. This became my way of taking care of my mother, because she was always so worried about my sister and money. I think I got lost somewhere along the way. But what never went away was this feeling of emptiness. I never felt filled up – until my eating disorder was out of control. People worried about me and had conversations about me. And I always would tell my mother that I hated the fact that she told everyone my business, but the truth of the matter was I felt my situation warranted as much attention and care as my sister. When I was in the hospital, people would just sit around all day and stay with me. They put aside whatever they were doing to take care of me. I felt I was important, and I liked it. But then it seemed to get out of hand, although I didn't really know it at the time, and I couldn't make it stop.

This all must sound so crazy and selfish. I feel so ashamed.

Carly: It doesn't sound crazy or selfish – just sad. In fact, it makes sense. As irrational a disorder as this is, it makes sense.

Jillian: I agree with Carly. It sounds as though you are now rediscovering who you are underneath your eating disorder. You are seeing yourself as someone who has an eating disorder rather than that being your only identity. You are beginning to question what your hunger was about and discovering your eating disorder was your attempt to fill a deep-seated need for attention and recognition.

Taylor: I can relate. I know what you mean about the attention. When I was really sick, it made people notice.

This is going to sound really nuts, but I used to love feeling like people envied me. I had this will-power they didn't have, and it made me feel so special – and it was mine, and no one could take it away.

Min: The empty feeling you guys describe sounds just like what I have felt so much on my life. Maybe it has something to do with my father traveling and being away all the time. But come to think of it, even when he was around, I felt it and worried about his next trip, and I longed for a closer relationship. Being at school and living so far away from my family seems to be stirring up some of the same feelings now. Maybe, in some ways, I'm trying to feel filled up with food.

Jillian: You all have effectively described the very common unsatisfied hunger that many of the young women in my previous groups have talked about. I'm not referring to physical hunger though. Let me explain.

For many young women with eating disorders, I have noticed their hungers were not all the same. They came in varying shapes and sizes, and they all originated from different places, but what was left standing from them was a deep underlying emptiness. There remained a void of some kind that they attempted to fill with their eating disorder. For some of them their hunger took on the form of deep emotional longing, which grew out of unresolved loss.

Min: What kind of loss do you mean?

Jillian: It could be for some, the loss of a parental figure through divorce, illness, addiction, or neglect. For others, the hollowness they experienced came as a result of their being ostracized by peers in junior high school. And for others, the void they carried was a representation of their ongoing search for meaning, purpose, and passion.

Anika: So, is what you are saying that these unresolved hungers actually feed the eating disorder.

Jillian: Yes, what many of these young women discovered was that they would either binge in an attempt to satiate feelings of emptiness or restrict in order to shrink away from the overwhelming feelings. What began for them as a subconscious and innocent attempt to cope with painful emotion, ended in behaviors that brought with them a whole host of their own negative consequences.

I would like to read you all an excerpt from ***Feeding the Hungry Heart*** by Geneen Roth to help explain further. Here she writes of her experience with Bulimia:

> Most striking to me was the connection between what I did to myself physically and its emotional correlation. I began to see I couldn't hate my body and ap-

preciate myself, that one was a reflection of the other. I saw that eating was not the problem. And by treating it as if it were – by dieting, depriving myself, hating my body – I was treating the symptoms without treating their cause. I saw that I needed to work from the inside out, from my feelings, my dreams, my angers, rather than the outside in, which began with my body.

Anika: Thanks so much for reading that – it makes so much sense to me. A quick change in perception can make all the difference.

Jillian: This is true. I think it is helpful if you all just sit with this for a while and see what comes up for you as you begin to process what Geneen Roth is expressing.

> *There is a short period of silence.*
> *Carly looks as if she has something she wants to say.*

Does anyone else have any thoughts?

Carly: I do, but it goes back to what Min was talking about – the topic of family and being away.
   I need to share something I haven't told anyone. I'm just beginning to realize it myself. I've been looking at colleges that are so far away. My parents have spent time and money taking me on all of these trips to see schools…and the truth of the matter is, part of me just wants to be at home and go to school close by. But then, I know my parents would start driving me crazy after a while and I would miss my friends. I don't get this. I've been away for years. For so long I wanted to be away with my friends. Now, why do I want to be home?

Jillian: I can understand why these questions are coming up for you now. And as uncomfortable as it is to ask them, I think they're coming up for you because you're paying attention to your needs and feelings. They are also coming up for you at a time when it is characteristic for someone your age to be asking them.

Carly: I'm not sure I understand what you mean.

Jillian: Maybe this will help.

Mary Pipher is well known for her writings on adolescence and the experience of extreme disconnection girls go through during this critical developmental period. She suggests that social norms and configurations of our culture force once-healthy, confident, free-thinking, and vociferous girls to be sentenced into silence and dependence. She explains that girls give up their individuality in attempt to secure themselves a place amongst their tenuous relationships with peers. It is at this time, as they are becoming more independent from their families, that they feel an increased need for psychological and emotional connection. With the stakes being so high, it becomes paramount for them to establish close bonds with their peers. In order to achieve this, they give up a part of themselves, that part which is the very essence of who they are – with all their likes, dislikes, and passions – to be able to fit in. Pipher explains it is this disconnection from who they really are that causes their emotional vulnerability. With this loss of self, they become prone to depression, addiction, and eating disorders as they are left searching for what has been lost.

Carly: Is this how my eating disorder developed?

Jillian: Not exactly, but I do think these developmental challenges are made that much more complicated by the dynamics at play with an eating disorder. In other words, perhaps your feelings of longing or dependency on your family have been magnified because of how intensely you feel your feelings, or because your underlying anxiety has made it more difficult for you to think about moving forward.

Carly: Yes, I can see that.

So, let me get this straight. My so called normal, complicated development becomes more complicated because I have an eating disorder.

Jillian: It can be more challenging.

I wonder what you feel may be able to help you in this situation?

Carly: Maybe talking about it with my parents some more. I mean there are so many options out there. I don't know why for so long I felt I was failing if I depended on my parents to much.

You know, I think my therapist might be able to help me understand this more.

Jillian: Great thought. If that is what you are comfortable with, try to do that.

Carly, I think you have discovered something very important from deep within you. I wish you luck as you continue to explore this further.

Carly: Thanks!

Jillian: Since we have talked here tonight about the topic of loss and moving on, and it seems to hold some difficulty for all of you, I would like to take a few moments to discuss the fact that pretty soon our group will be ending. Although we have two more weeks left, I am wondering what this feels like for all of you?

Taylor: Wow that sucks!

I don't know where all the time went. I remember thinking I probably wasn't going to make it to too many groups because I didn't think I'd have a ride. Now, I wouldn't miss one.

Jillian: I am glad you have been able to connect so well, Taylor.

Carly: I'm saddened by this fact.

For the first time in my two years of therapy, I feel like I understand so much more about me and my eating disorder. Not that it's any easier, it's just different, and I swear it is because of all of you.

Jillian: Carly, it is wonderful the self discovery that has been occurring for you. Remember, even as our time together ends you can take tools that you have learned here and use them in your life.

Carly: I guess you are right.

Min: I have to say, I have learned so much here and I wish I could keep coming and learning more.

I feel like this is the best education I have received in a long time.

Stephanie: I agree with Min. Do you think there's any way we could keep meeting? Even once a month or something just to see how everyone is doing?

Jillian: It's understandable that thinking about our group coming to an end is painful, scary, disappointing, and uncertain. You all have done such hard work and have opened your hearts to one another and taken incredible risks together. You have reached out to each other and eased the pain that accompanies emptiness and isolation. You have felt connections in here that have added new meaning to your lives. I know this is difficult. But I also know that within this newfound meaning, you have made room not only for seeds to grow, but entire gardens.

I have so much faith and belief in all of you. You all have shown great strength here.

Stephanie, I understand what you are saying about meeting once a month to keep in some contact could be helpful. What I have found works well for many young women is to end at week nine and then have a kind of reunion in a few months to see where everyone is at.

Is this something everyone would like to do?

Stephanie: Absolutely!

Taylor: I'll be here, even if I have to hitch a ride.

Min: I would truly be grateful for that.

Carly: Yes, let's do that!

Jillian: Okay We will be planning this more during our last groups together.

One more important piece I would like you all to think about is the fact that although we may not be physically meeting every week, the connections and bonds that have occurred here will be a part of you for the rest of your lives. This is another reason why group therapy can be so beneficial in recovery.

Before we end tonight, I feel like it would be helpful and appropriate to share with all of you something personal from me.

I would like to share with you an excerpt that I included in a letter I had written to one of the girls who had been in my groups for years off and on. She struggled very hard in her recovery. During her last hospitalization I wrote her this letter, from which I will read you a small part that I hope will help you all find meaning for yourselves and your lives.

It's amazing how the paper still smells the same to me as the day I wrote this to her.

> When someone is in the throes of an eating disorder, life can feel as though it is becoming smaller and smaller, until there is little left besides the thoughts, the behaviors, and the consequences of the disorder. In time, what you initially relied upon as a defense to cope with an inner hunger only deepens the void. Soon, it becomes harder to embrace the ideals, the people, and the dreams that were at one time so important.
>
> Although difficult, try to challenge yourself to reconnect with those aspects of your life which at one time made you feel excited to be alive. Pursue relationships you think will bring the promise of friendship. Learn who your heroes are. Soak up the moments that bring you joy. And when there's sadness, discover how these tears may fit into the bigger plan for your life. When emotions have been so overwhelming, it is easy to lose sight of the fact that our bodies are made to be able to feel feelings, to cry when we are sad and laugh when we're happy. Be confident that, in allowing yourself to have these experiences, you are deepening your capacity to live life to its fullest, and you are connecting with your authentic self.

Stephanie: That is beautiful.

This may not be appropriate to ask, but has this client recovered?

Jillian: Actually, she lost her fight with Anorexia and she did die. It was one month after I gave her the letter.

Although she struggled for many years and the outcome of her recovery was not what she deserved, I learned so very much about just how powerful an eating disorder can be. It might sound very strange, but in her pain and darkest times, she became a teacher without ever realizing it.

Stephanie: I can't believe I am crying and I don't even know her. It's just what you said is so beautiful.

Jillian: I think it's wonderful that you can show this emotion. This is very painful to hear. The reality of mortality in relation to an eating disorder is very terrifying and even more when you are struggling with Anorexia or Bulimia.

It is important to remember that everyone's story is different and each of you have the ability to allow your recovery to be what you want and need.

Are there any other thoughts or concerns on this difficult topic before we end our evening here tonight?

Min: I just wanted to say, I had no idea how serious eating disorders are.

Taylor: I agree. I mean for years people threw the death card at me saying "If you keep losing weight, your heart could stop and you could die." I have to say I never took that seriously. But for some reason listening to you, Jillian, explain what you did and knowing that this girl died anyway, kind of really freaks me out. I guess what I mean is, I believe in the true dangers now.

Jillian: Well, my intention is not to instill fear in any of you. But, unfortunately death can become a reality for some who continuously struggle with an eating disorder over periods of time. I think hearing of the experiences of others that may not have had "happy endings" is an opportunity for others to learn. So if possible, learn from this story of my client.

Carly: I agree with you.

This might sound really cold and harsh, but I don't mean it to be. Listening to all of this, kind of empowered me. I realized when you were talking about her that I did not want that to be me. This experience tonight kind of gave me a spark to make sure I win this battle.

Jillian: Carly, I am so pleased for you and I don't think what you said was cold at all. It seems like very intelligent thinking. Keep up your fight, however long it takes. You have a wonderful will.

On a much more optimistic note, I just wanted to mention something about next week's group. You all have done so much work here, I realize I keep saying this, but it is true. Because of this I would like to do something a little different.

As an exercise to help promote each of your self-esteem and recognition, I would like you to bring something in to the group that you are proud of. This could be a talent of some kind, something you have made or written in the past, a story of something you did, a photograph of a place or a person in your life you are proud of, or you could play music if you play an instrument….or even sing. I'd like to leave it up to each of you.

I'm looking forward to experiencing this with everyone.

I will offer you all some inspiration before we part for this evening. My intention is for each of you to find tonight's *Words of Hope* helpful.

> When a field lies barren for a while, and then it is finally seeded, it is that much richer for the long wait. And the fruit it now bears can prosper in abundance.

Enjoy your week everyone – Spring is in the air! Until our next time together, be well.

Week Eight

Culture & Values

Throughout the group forums I have facilitated, the issue of **culture and values** seems to be a struggle for many, while impacting their eating disorder on many levels.

The female roles in our culture have changed, and continue to change over the years. Many of the girls have discussed our cultural emphasis on lookism, perfectionism, and the idea of women being objectified for many reasons, including selling products.

It is also apparent that our culture focuses great emphasis on outcomes and what we produce, not our inner worth. Society sends messages that reflect the idea that females are to take up as little space as possible; physically, emotionally, and mentally.

Together, these unrealistic ideals reinforce the insecurities of young women. It is understandable why many may feel they must look a certain way and act a certain way. This dysfunctional standard also reinforces the idea of being busy and productive, constantly doing for others, yet having no worth.

Our society is also guilty of creating confusion around values. This happens because of the great societal emphasis on productivity and less emphasis on family values. Many parents have expressed to me the belief, that in working at high demanding jobs that often consume great amounts of their time, they can offer their children all the opportunities they deserve. When in reality these young girls need opportunities and moments within their family unit to become truly healthy and successful adults.

Many of the young women who develop eating disorders or

have body image issues, and have parents whose employment requires them to be less present in the home, often feel a great sense of disconnection, isolation, and loneliness. This then creates a forced dependence on their peers and relationships prematurely. These young women are searching for the acceptance from their circle of friends that they may be lacking within their family. These dynamics often develop into difficult situations, leading to increased anxiety, fear, and loss of control, which then reinforces their eating disorder behaviors and can affect the recovery process. It becomes easy, to then recognize, the results of our society lacking healthy culture and values and how it affects young girls.

Managing Culture and Values

Over the years, I have found it to be beneficial to promote and encourage in young females a sense of empathy, compassion, and understanding, while promoting their own self esteem. In doing so, these females are more capable of taking the time to listen to others with an open heart, which can be empowering. It allows them to view the world with an open mind instead of the closed mind that mimics the eating disorder and other rigid thoughts. In contrast, I also believe it is imperative to teach **media literacy**, and help young women recognize that they can follow the ideals that feel comfortable to them and not what society or a culture may be demanding of them.

Many of the girls have expressed to me, that when they have been able to achieve living this way, they feel they have options and are not "so stuck". When they are able to develop this strength, whether in the recovery process or beyond, they are better able to resist falling victim to our society's misleading ideas of expectations and values.

What unhealthy messages are you receiving from our society? Have you ever explored the effects that these messages have had on your life and your eating disorder? During recovery you will have an opportunity to develop an internal filter that recognizes these delusional cultural messages and therefore help you resist being affected by them. I understand at this point it may not seem possible, but as you will notice in this Week all the girls in some way, even subtly, are becoming empowered by discussing their angst about their need for acceptance and the onslaught of negative messages we receive as females. I am sure you also have a wonderful, intelligent voice that deserves to be heard related to this issue of culture and values. Allow yourself to speak up when you are ready!

> Over the last several years, my friends have been like my surrogate family. They've been there for decisions about clothes, relationships, or whatever. Looking back, I feel as though I pushed my family away because that's what I was supposed to do.
>
> *– Carly*

Jillian: Welcome back everyone. I would like us to begin as soon as everyone is ready, so we can utilize the time we have these last few weeks together.

> *The girls are standing up talking with each other engaging in casual, light-hearted conversations.*

Let's all find a comfortable seat and begin.

What has been happening for each of you since we were last together?

Carly: Is it Okay if I just kind of dive in?

Jillian: I think that seems fine.

Carly: I have so many things I want to talk about, and I'm so glad it's finally Tuesday. But I can't believe we only have one more week left…and that gives me such an ache in the pit of my stomach.

Remember last week when I was talking about how I might not want to go so far away to college? Well, I finally brought it up with my parents. They were initially kind of shocked and worried. They thought I was feeling this way because things were going badly with my eating disorder and I want to be close to home. But I assured them this wasn't the case. I just wanted to be close to my family…and even my dog. I think they're beginning to understand. So, in a few weeks, we are going to start checking into local colleges that have really good swim teams. And I'm thinking I might want to go into social work or something related.

I'm starting to get really excited.

Jillian: That's great, Carly. It must be quite a relief to have this out in the open now. Listening to you talk about this struggle, about how it can be okay to be dependent on your family, brings up a question I would like to ask you. Would that be Okay?

Carly: Sure.

Jillian: I was wondering, do you think there is any similarity between the way you interact with your family and the way your peers relate to theirs?

Carly: Well, in some ways I feel as though I'm coming full circle. Over the last several years, I think my friends have been like my surrogate family. They're always there for decisions about clothes, relationships, family, or whatever. Looking back, it almost feels as though I pushed my family away because that's what I was supposed to do – and it's what everyone else was doing. Well, don't get me wrong, they also annoyed the hell out of me at times, and I wanted them far away. But I felt I had to push them away because this was the way of the world – no questions asked – might as well do it sooner rather than later.

Jillian: It sounds like what you are saying is, you almost forced yourself to emotionally distance your family, because you thought there was an implicit cultural expectation to do so. Where do you think that message came from?

Carly: Everywhere. I mean when I was younger, if I was invited to a sleepover and I didn't want to go because I wanted to be at home, my friends thought I was weird or something. If you were having problems with friends and you talked to your parents about it instead of the other girls, they thought this was weird too. And I remember when I started liking boys, if I told my friends I talked to my parents about boys, they thought I was crazy. And now, I feel like I'm supposed to go away and begin establishing a life separate from my family.

Jillian: Carly, you have done amazing offering the group a clear picture of the pressures our culture and its values can have on each of you as you have been growing up.

I wonder, do you think this sense of forced independence had any impact on your eating disorder?

Carly: I guess I don't really see the connection. Do you?

Jillian: I do.

You describe this dynamic where teens embrace their peers more and more as they distance themselves from family, and in this culture this is viewed as almost a developmental expectation. Within the book *The Second Family*, Dr. Ron Taffel talks about this phenomenon. He explains how kids at a younger and younger age are all embracing their peers as their first family. In turn, their nuclear family then becomes secondary. He explains this has happened, in part, as a result of the excessive demands placed on parents these days. These demands force them into having busier schedules and being less available at home. In response, children and teens gravitate more toward one another, and they use technology – mostly cell phones and computers – as a way of maintaining and solidifying their connection with each other.

Stephanie: What kind of impact do you think all of this has on us emotionally that could impact our eating disorders?

Week Eight: Culture & Values   177

Jillian: I would like to turn the question around and ask you all what you think.

I want to hear your views.

Min: Although I know we're talking about a different culture than my own, I definitely think this "forced independence" has had an impact on me. I now understand I've used food as a substitute for connection with family. And I think my family sees my independence as a necessity. They think if I stray from this path, I won't have a chance to be successful in a competitive economy.

Jillian: Min, this is valuable insight.

Let me take what Min is saying a little further.

There are experts in the field of eating disorders who believe eating disorders exist because they are a symptom of what is ailing our larger culture and less of our individual psychopathology. Although we may be personally impacted, they theorize that the root cause of this problem can be found amidst a historical and cultural perspective.

Min: Could you explain more?

Yes, I have this book titled *Eating Disorders and Cultures in Transition*. The author is Richard Gordon and he explains this:

> The fact that eating disorders occur overwhelmingly in women, however, cannot be fully comprehended without addressing the critical transitions in female identity that have characterized the late twentieth century in industrialized or rapidly industrializing societies. As women have moved in increasing numbers into spheres of education and work around the globe, expectation for achievement and performance have sometimes conflicted sharply with insistent demands for traditional postures of dependency and submissiveness as well as a renewed cult of physical appearance that has been fed by corporate forces. The result of these contradictory pressures has been, for many, an enhanced sense of personal uncertainty and

self-doubt, along with an increased sense of power-lessness.

Min: Wow, that really sums it up.

Jillian: Yes, Gordon's viewpoint reflects a widely held, yet sometimes controversial belief, that eating disorders occur within cultures undergoing dramatic social and political change. As a result of these changes, women experience confusion and conflict over their roles within the family and within the workforce. This confusion then creates an identity crisis, which is reflected in our bodies. Eating disorders are seen as a metaphor, as a symbol of society's greater turmoil.

Min: I really do agree with this. It seems that this idea that this excerpt exhibits is also demonstrated with younger girls, just on a different level.

Jillian: Absolutely true, very similar to what Carly was discussing.

Stephanie: I'm not sure if this relates, but for me, I guess my eating disorder was kind of a way of "putting the brakes on" independence in some ways. I mean it was definitely a cry for attention and recognition because I always felt so forgotten about, but in some ways I think I needed it because the world felt so unsafe. I watched my peers with their parties in high school, their boyfriends, and their talk about who was hooking up with whom, their competitiveness and back stabbing. I think I just got scared and overwhelmed. I felt I couldn't rely on my mother because she was already too stressed. Her world was not really one I wanted to enter into. I guess I insulated myself by not eating.

Jillian: This is definitely related. Is there more, Stephanie?

Stephanie: Yes, I know I'm doing a lot of talking, but I was wondering if I could talk about something that happened to me this week that really bothered me.

Jillian: Sure, this is what our time together is for.

Stephanie: I've realized since the group started, I've been trying to make more of an effort to spend time on campus on the weekends – to get more involved. I stayed on campus this past weekend, and I was over at a friend's dorm, where a bunch of girls and guys were watching TV They were watching some cop show.

There are two male cops at a crime scene where a young woman was recently murdered, and they're examining her body for evidence. And they are talking about her like she's an object or a piece of meat or something. I know its TV, but it really bothered me. And then one cop says to the other one, "It's always such a disappointment when such a pretty girl has shoddy underwear." The girl is dead! I was so angry, and I'm thinking, "Gee, she should have planned better for this." So, even when you're dead you can't let your guard down! You have to be perfect.

Why did I feel so personally violated and disrespected? What made it that much worse was I couldn't tell anyone how I felt because they thought the comment was humorous.

Jillian: That sounds very difficult.

I'm wondering what it means to you to feel like you have to have your "guard" up?

Stephanie: Well, it seems that as females we are always being examined or judged or rated in some way. It just reinforces that whole perspective, that we have to be perfect, that it's what's on the outside that counts.

Carly: I understand exactly what you mean, Stephanie. I had one of those cringe moments a couple of nights ago.

For the most part, I've been making an effort not to read fashion magazines or watch TV. I used to be a magazine and reality show junky, but they're so triggering, and they always left me feeling so bad about myself. But the other night, in a weaker moment, I was flipping through the channels, and there were three different makeover shows going on at the same time. I couldn't believe it.

Taylor: How are they triggering for you?

Carly: Because, when I watch reality shows I compare myself to everyone! And all the girls are so damn gorgeous and skinny! When I would watch with my boyfriend, I'd imagine that he would be fantasizing about being with them instead of me – even though he thinks I'm crazy.

Jillian: Carly, I wonder what else about these reality shows bothers you.

Carly: They just reinforce the whole notion that to be happy we have to fit in with the ideal standards, and if we can't, we are to be pitied and reconstructed.

Taylor: I'm totally shocked you guys compare yourselves to people on TV, because I do the same thing. Actually, I compare myself to everyone.

In the beginning, before our group first started, I was so worried about what everyone would look like. I was afraid I'd be fatter than everyone else.

I feel really bad about saying this, but my best friend is on a diet – and I'm glad for her, because she's really unhappy about her weight – but selfishly, I don't want her to lose weight. I like feeling smaller then her. In fact, I like being smaller than my boyfriend too. I don't think I could go out with anyone unless they were a lot bigger than me.

Anika: If I may say something, I think men in this culture are threatened by women with larger builds. I think they're worried we will be too opinionated or outspoken and we'll threaten their masculinity. We're supposed to be the ones that never get too angry, who keep the peace, just smooth things over and move on.

Carly: Yeah, or they won't be able to dominate us so easily!

Jillian: Wow, you girls have so much to say about these issues of our culture and society.

Let's talk a little more about this idea of culture. You all seem to be saying, in your own way, that because you are female, and you have grown up the way you have, there are specific expectations on you. What are these expectations?

Taylor: To be beautiful. If you are chubby or fat, you are less likable.

Stephanie: I feel we all have to look alike. To be different, or diverse, or not mainstream, is to be less valued. Don't be too smart or you'll stand out and be ridiculed, and don't be too stupid or you'll stand out.

Jillian: Anything else?

Carly: I agree with what Anika was saying about how women cannot be too assertive, or men, and even other women, seem to be threatened.

Anika: I'm not sure if this is exactly what you are looking for, but one thing I've experienced about men in this country is that they think just because you go out with them, you're going to have sex with them.

Jillian: Many of these observations all of you are making about our culture, how we perceive ourselves and each other, and how we expect others to respond to us, stem from the way we are portrayed in the media. Women are frequently portrayed as mindless objects used to sell products, rather than as thinking and feeling individuals. We are often presented as lustful and over-sexualized creatures that will stop at nothing until we get what we want. And we are shown as being easily dominated and humiliated by men.

An eager expression appears on Min's face
Min, you look like you want to say something. Is there anything you want to share about this topic of culture and media?

Min: Yes I do. I was thinking about where all this pressure on thinness and physical perfection might originate. It seems hard to know for sure where it all gets started, because it just permeates.

I haven't spent a lot of time at home in a while, but I was talking with a friend of mine from Seoul recently, and she was telling me that liposuction surgeons have sprung up there everywhere. And now the latest craze is diet powders, pills, cellulite creams, and other herbal products that promise to "shed" pounds. I was recently reading that in Japan they're advertising all of these products which supposedly promote facial slimming. There are signs everywhere with pictures of women complaining that their faces are too fat.

How does all of this get started?

Jillian: Great question. Similar to the excerpt by Gordon I read to you earlier, a lot of research is being done to try to answer these questions. So far, they're seeing a higher presence of eating disorders and body image dissatisfaction in countries that are more westernized or modernized. They are also seeing them, to a large degree, in counties where there has been a dramatic change in the roles and expectations of women. It is important to note that what was thought of at one time as a white, upper class phenomenon is now becoming a global issue, one crossing all social, economic, and cultural ties.

We have spent many weeks together exploring some of the cognitive and emotional parallels women with eating disorders experience, and we have examined some of the biochemical, psychological, and social factors that influence eating disorders. Yet until this point, we have not looked at the correlation between eating disorders and cultures, and I feel to miss this would be like looking at the incidence of global warming without it's connection to geography or politics.

Min: This is interesting, yet very disturbing.

Anika: I agree. All this talk is so depressing. It makes me feel so helpless.

Jillian: Understandably so, but I do believe there are things you can do that can make a difference, and, in fact, all of you have made a great beginning here this evening. You have opened your own eyes to the true impact of this problem and to the factors that influence it. From this knowledge and awareness, you can make decisions about how much you want to get involved to effect change. There are avenues to become active – either on a personal level or a more political level – if you have the interest.

Anika: Do you have any suggestion on doing this effectively?

Jillian: Yes. If you have the energy, you can raise awareness by starting discussion groups on campus or in organizing efforts to make changes within the fashion industry toward how women are portrayed. **It can be very therapeutic and healing to direct some of your energy into activism.**

As we continue, I would like to share with you something that may offer all of you some comfort that others are acknowledging and fighting against the damage societal and cultural factors are having on young women.

Have all of you heard of "Take our Daughters to Work Day"? This day, now a national event, started because of a collaborative effort between Carol Gilligan and Marie Wilson, the two leaders of the Harvard Project On Women's Psychology and Girl's Development, and The Ms. Foundation. Their collaboration began as a conversation over their mutual concern for what was happening to girls as they moved into adolescence. In their book they reflect on this concern.

> As diverse as we were, and as able as we had become, each of us had walked a similar path: We all remembered an early time of feeling brave and free, bold and full of self pride; we all moved through a voice-silencing, spirit-silencing transition as our bodies evolved, as our relationship with our mothers changed, as we developed sexual feelings, and as the world began to see us in women's bodies.

I personally feel this clearly describes what happens as we develop from young girls into women.

The wonderful thing about this is what developed from a

conversation about their mutual concern for girls, later became an idea to launch a consciousness raising campaign called "A Girl Is Watching; What is She Learning?" Their intent was to air public service announcements with this slogan after commercials and television shows that portrayed women as unrealistic and inauthentic. Their idea then merged in the nineties with a speech given by ABC anchorman Peter Jennings at an AIDS commemorative service. As part of his address, he read an essay written by his daughter. Jennings had recognized his own daughter's voice "by taking her to work." The suggestion of recognizing a young girl's voice, by putting her in an influential setting such as the workplace, took hold and later became a national event.

Taylor: I know this is totally off the topic from what you just said, kind of, but how the hell is it possible not to compare yourself to other girls. I mean, I feel like I get messages every day from friends, family, TV, and radio that I must do this for my own survival.

Jillian: I am glad you brought this up, Taylor, and it does fit in with what we are talking about.

Girls in recovery have told me that what has been really useful to them is to try to approach other girls, no matter how attractive they are, with the same spirit of compassion that they try to approach themselves with. And they have found that if they are unable to extend feelings of compassion to others, then, at the very least, they try approaching them with a stance of curiosity. In other words, we have the habit of assuming we know what someone is like by the way they look. **Yet if you were to approach a stranger with a curiosity about their lives, rather than a set of preconceived beliefs, you would feel less threatened by them. You would also be helping to change our cultural emphasis on looks.**

Taylor: That is quite a "take charge of your own destiny" thought – it's kind of cool I guess.

Carly: I recently came across two quotes by Mahatma Gandhi that have made a big impact on me, in a way that not many others have, it may help here for us this evening. They have stuck with me, and they keep replaying in my head. I think they will help give me the strength I need to keep going in my recovery. They're really simple.

One says: "Be the change that you want to see in the world." And the other: "A small body of determined spirits fired up by an unquenchable faith in their mission can alter the course of history."

Jillian: These are wonderful quotes, and so appropriate. Thank you for sharing them with us.

Anika: I love those.

Mahatma Gandhi was so brilliant and has always been special to my family. Thanks for offering those, Carly.

Carly: You are very welcome. I hope they offer you all something like they offer me!

Jillian: Thank you all for sharing this evening. I have to tell you, I am truly honored to have been witness to the insight that travels around this circle that we sit together in.

On that note, I think now would be a wonderful time to do what we discussed last week. Just to refresh everyone's memory, last week I told all of you I wanted to give each of you the opportunity to share with the group a side of yourself we don't usually have the good fortune of seeing. I asked you to bring in a part of you that you are proud of.

Does anyone want to share what they have brought?

Carly: Could I please go first? I'm feeling really inspired after our discussion today.

Jillian: I think that is fine. What have you brought in to share?

Carly: This feels really strange.

I didn't bring anything, I am going to sing a song I heard a while ago that has always really touched me in a very powerful way.

My voice is rusty, and it's been a while, so bear with me.

Carly stands in the middle of the group's circle.

The song is by Wilson Phillips. It's called **Hold On**.

Carly sings. Her choice of a song is ideal: it is an updated version of Emerson's "Most of the shadows of this life are caused by standing in one's own sunshine." She starts tentatively, but her delivery gathers strength and dignity. Her listeners are swept away.

When she finishes, there is an extended moment of silence.

Stephanie: I didn't know you could sing! You have a real talent! Your voice is beautiful, and that's always been one of my favorite songs.

Is there a reason you chose that song?

Carly: When I first heart heard the song, it really struck me, especially when it says "break free from your chains." I felt like the song was giving me permission to break free from my eating disorder.

Taylor: Holy crap, I love that song, but I never thought about it that way before.

Cool insight.

Anika: Have you ever done any recording?

Carly: No. I've had some parts in school plays and once for a Summer theatre production, but nothing serious.

Taylor: You should. You have a kick-ass voice. I mean you could be in a band!

Carly: I have always had a secret fantasy of being in a band.

Jillian: Carly, that was beautiful, and the lyrics were so inspiring.

It was wonderful to hear many of your responses to Carly. This demonstrates the true connection you all have to one another.

Thank you.

Does anyone else have something they want to share?

Min: I do. I haven't done any painting or drawing since being away from home – it makes me too homesick – but I brought in a painting I did a few years ago of one of my favorite water gardens.

Min uncovers a medium size canvas painted in soothing pastels.
For many years, I've painted greeting cards of gardens or flowers and sold them to people I know, or just give them as presents. In fact, it was in this group that I started thinking about doing them again and including in them some inspirational sayings. Actually, I came across a quote the other day that I think will be perfect for my first one. It was written by Anais Nin. Here is my painting…and I'd like to read the quote for you all.

And the day came when the risk it took to remain tight in the bud was more painful than the risk it took to blossom.

I don't know when I'm going to have time to work on it, but I'm really excited about it.

Stephanie: Min, the quote is extraordinary, and so is your artwork. I think you could really do something with your idea.
I wish I could paint or draw. I love water colors, but whenever I try to use them, I get so frustrated.

Min: Thank you, Stephanie. Just remember, frustration can alter creativity. Try to let yourself be creative without judgment.
This is the one area of my life where I feel carefree.

Carly: You know, just your painting alone is inspirational. The colors are so touching – it's like they reach my soul, and nowadays, Asian artwork – just about anything from placemats to bamboo shades – is so popular. That's not the only reason to do it. You're good at it. You have a gift and you totally light up when talking about it.

Min: Thank you so much!

Jillian: What extraordinary talent and sensitivity there is in this room.

Min, thank you for sharing this beautiful creative side with our group.

Who would like to have a turn next?

Taylor: Actually, I brought in something I just finished making this week in my art class.

We're doing ceramics, which I've never done before, and I really didn't think I'd like it, but I like working with the clay. It was so nice just to be able to turn off my head and do something with my hands. I found it relaxing and soothing, and when I'm angry, it's something to pound. I was trying to figure out what to make, and I couldn't think of anything. Then, all of a sudden, I got this image of Elisabeth in my head. In fact, I've been thinking about her all week. I didn't really even try to do this. It's like my hands just did it. I made a sculpture of Elisabeth with her baby girl, and that's what I brought in.

*Nervously, Taylor reaches into a brown paper bag
and reveals the sculpture.*

I'm actually thinking of giving it to her. Do you think that would be Okay?

Jillian: I think that would be very kind of you. I will talk to her so maybe you both can connect in the near future.

What did your teacher think of your work?

Taylor: She said she thought I had a hidden talent and I should take more sculpting or pottery classes. She told me about one that will be starting up soon, but I'm not sure if I would have the money to do it. Besides, maybe I just got lucky with this one.

Anika: No, I think there is more to it than just luck. That's an amazing figure, and I think you have found a way to channel some of all those powerful feelings you have inside.

Taylor: Thanks.

Min: Taylor, I think the sculpture demonstrates the beauty of human emotion. I don't believe that is something just anybody can do.

Taylor: That's nice to hear.

Jillian: Taylor, I am delighted you have found such a creative resource to channel the energy that comes with your feelings – good for you!

Anika or Stephanie, would either of you like to share?

Anika: I will, but Taylor, try not to doubt your ability.

I don't have the talent that all of you do, so I decided to bring in a picture of my great-grandmother, because to me she is a symbol of what's really important in life. To me, she represents strength and courage.

Anika reaches into her purse
and takes out a black and white photo.

My parents told me she was part of a movement in India that followed World War I. This was when Mahatma Gandhi organized a movement of passive resistance against Great Britain. My great-grandmother held a job in public office, and as an act of rebellion against colonial repression, she walked off her job – as Gandhi had instructed. As a result, she and her children, one of whom was my grandfather, later overcame extreme hardships in the times that followed. I like to think I have some small part of her inside of me.

Min: I think you have more than just a small part of her inside of you. In fact, you really look like her.

Anika: Thanks, Min.

Some of the people in my family don't ever talk about her, because I think in some ways they're uncomfortable with a woman being such a strong and individual thinker. I've really had to pull information from them.

They don't even realize I have this picture.

Carly: I can't believe you're somehow connected with Gandhi.

Stephanie: That's such a fascinating story. Anika, do you think your great-grandmother actually got to hear Gandhi speak or meet him?

Anika: I'm not really sure.

Taylor: Nothing like that has ever happened in my boring stupid family.

Can I see the picture up close?

Anika: Sure.

Taylor: Wow she really is beautiful. Her eyes look magical. I really love all the jewelry.

Anika: Yes, she is dressed in her classic Indian attire for this picture after she was able to prevail.

Taylor: So cool!

Jillian: Anika, I am sure you do have talents, you may have not discovered yet. But what you brought in to our group is very appropriate. I think it is wonderful that you have somebody in your family that you can gain strength from – even though you never met her. The bonds that exist between families can be truly amazing.

Stephanie, would you like to share something with all of us?

Stephanie: Sure, I didn't know what to bring in, so I decided even though it wasn't finished yet I'd show you the scrapbook I've been making for my sister. It's taken many years, and my plan is to give it to her when she turns ten. She has no idea I saved all this stuff – pictures she's made me, her ribbons from dance recitals, projects from school, old photographs…I even saved a piece of her first baby blanket.

Stephanie takes a flat box from under her chair and removes the album.

Carly: Wow, this is a masterpiece. Does she even know you've been working on it?

Stephanie: No. I started it a long time ago when we first discovered she was sick. It was my way of being able to hold onto every little piece of her. My mother doesn't even know I have it. She'd probably think it was a little strange.

Anika: I can really see you put your heart and soul into it. And the artwork is so beautiful and detailed.

Stephanie: I've been lucky, because as I've been developing it, the art of scrapbooking has really taken off. It used to be much harder to find fancy paper and little decorations. It's actually been really soothing to work on it when I'm upset about something.

Min: You are very artistic, and your sister is going to be so amazed.

I'd love to learn how to do this. Maybe I could even incorporate some of the technique into my greeting cards.

Stephanie: It's easy. I'd be happy to teach you.

Jillian: Stephanie, what an absolutely wonderful way to celebrate your sister's life.

Stephanie: Thank you. I wish you all could meet her. She's an incredible person, and she'd really love you guys.

Jillian: Stephanie, thank you for bringing something so important to you and allowing us to learn more about your sister.

I want to offer sincere gratitude to all of you. Sitting here as the sun begins to set, watching each of you share such deeply personal sides of yourselves has been such a gift. I am deeply moved by what I have experienced here tonight with everyone. You are all unique and special in so many ways. Thank you for everything you have and continue to offer this group.

The setting sun casts its warm soothing glow through the window onto the group.

Unfortunately, next week is our last week together. I think at that time we could arrange a time, at the end of the Summer, for us to come back together. Coming together after some time passes will be an opportunity to reconnect with one another, check in on how everyone is doing, and look at any challenges that might have come up for you over the Summer, as well as triumphs. This plan is consistent with my belief that women and girls need communities of others for support, places where they can gather together periodically in order to strengthen themselves or rediscover who they are.

Stephanie: I feel so relieved right now.

Carly: Yes, me too. No matter what I have going on, I would never pass up spending and evening with all of you!

Jillian: I think it is wonderful that you both are able to recognize and acknowledge that you are comfortable with this plan for our special coming together group.

We have done a great amount of work here this evening. I hope each of you can give yourself credit for being so present and for all the discussions we have had together.

Before we part, I would like to offer all of you a gift (a. k. a. *Words of Hope*) for this evening.

> When one person who is uncomfortable stops to question how things are being done, it can open up so many possibilities for others.

Week Nine

Moving Forward

Although moving forward is not a core struggle, I do consider it a struggle in recovery. In my years of facilitating groups, I have found as an eating disorder group is ending, the members begin to anticipate not only the loss of the group, but also moving forward, and the changes that may occur with that.

For many, when a situation ends or they experience a change or loss within a relationship, it can bring up other unresolved losses. This then places more stress on someone when they are already vulnerable because of their own recovery.

It is very challenging for many of the girls as a group meets for the final time. This is because many have relied on the support of the group to help them cope. Now this support is ending or changing and they many need more support. For the young women struggling with an eating disorder, this experience of loss can truly affect where they are in their recovery process.

Managing Moving Forward

Prior to the eating disorder groups ending I have found it helpful for many of the girls to use support from those who may understand them and that they can trust. This then creates a foundation for them as they anticipate moving on. During the last few weeks of the groups, I often remind the girls to acknowledge what others in the group may be feeling. This not only helps them realize they are not alone (because others may be having a hard time with the transition, too), but also helps them become aware of the feelings they may be experiencing.

Whether it is a group ending, a relationship changing, or some other loss is endured, extra support may be necessary during this time. As many girls work through their recovery and discover more about themselves, their wants and needs, it becomes easier to have the proper support in place. This is ideal for continuing their journey of recovery in a healthy direction.

I am wondering what you may be feeling at this point in the book. You have gotten to know all the members of the group as you have been a witness to their trials and triumphs of their own recoveries. Allow yourself extra support at this time if you sense you need it. For the group members their time together is ending, yet for you, you are able at any time to go back and re-experience moments that may be beneficial for you from these 9 weeks. As you read this Week about moving forward, whether you are leaving an inpatient facility, or experiencing life changes, the intention is to offer you the encouragement you may need at whatever crossroads you may be facing. Trust that as your recovery evolves, the ability to move forward in your life will happen with more ease.

I have learned so much from the people in this group. I wish we could go on meeting forever. We could share all of each other's milestones and challenges together.

– Anika

Jillian: Before we begin, I want to let everyone know that I have decided to leave open the windows a little this evening. The air is so warm, fresh, and calming today. I find the energy of this time of day very powerful.

Welcome to our last group – for a while.

As I was getting ready to begin my day this morning, I caught myself reflecting about this group. Looking back upon the journey we have traveled together over the past several weeks, I realized most of the work we have done together has been about becoming your authentic selves.

There are many well-known authors who have written about the concept of an **authentic self**. One in particular came to my mind today. Joan Borensyko refers to this term as being "self-full"-filled with who we are. Please correct me if I'm wrong, but I think each of you has had the opportunity to discover how to listen to your inner voice, to be quiet and reflective. You may have also learned to pay attention to your feelings and to use them to guide your decisions. It seems that this group has realized that behind each of your emotions there are also needs. You are all slowly learning to communicate those needs to others. Remember, by discovering who you really are you will develop core strength, an inner compass, to guide you as you move through life.

At this very moment, I wish you all could change places with me. What I am trying to say is, I wish each of you could sit where I am and see yourself and your growth the way I do. You have done such hard work. It is truly amazing to me.

Now that you have heard my thoughts, I wonder how each of you are doing this evening?

Anika: For me, I can't believe we're not going to see each other for awhile. Tuesday nights aren't going to be the same without all of you. It's going to be so strange, and I don't know exactly what I'll do without the group.

As far as my eating goes, I've had a pretty good week. It's been a little harder than usual because I have a difficult time with change. I think I've been eating more to deal with the anxiety of not knowing what's ahead.

Jillian: It is amazing how much you've learned about yourself and how you are now able to identify what is behind your eating.

I don't know too many people who do well with change or transition in life, and although we may acknowledge this on some levels, I don't think we adequately prepare ourselves for the true impact. For example, when major events occur in our lives – trips to new places, a move, marriage, a new job, and illness, the loss of someone close – most of us don't truly acknowledge the full impact that they can have on our lives. And if we do, it's usually our expectation, and the expectation of those around us, that life should go on as normal. We aren't really given permission to openly acknowledge the true and ongoing impact of these transitions as we need to. After a while, it seems people stop checking in with us to see how we are coping, and, perhaps we do, too.

Anika: For me our group ending is similar to the major events you just spoke of.

Jillian: Yes, in fact I am viewing the group like one of those transitions.

You are all not only dealing with preparation for Summer, reconnecting with family, a new job, some of you are thinking about plans for college. And, in addition, you have spent the last eight weeks considering your thoughts, feelings, and what goes into them. You have spent time looking at the possibilities of what life could be like without your eating disorder, and this is a departure from the way you looked at life before. This is a change. Try to be especially compassionate with yourselves.

Anika, do you have any definite plans for your Summer?

Anika: I'm going to be away for a few weeks with my aunt and uncle doing some traveling, and then I'll be starting the internship in a law office sometime in late Summer or early Fall.

Jillian: How do you feel about these plans?

Anika: I'm nervous and excited.

I am planning to journal a lot if things get crazy with my health and body obsessed aunt. Yet, I cannot wait for this internship.

Jillian: It is inspiring that you have a plan to keep yourself safe and healthy if things become difficult. Best wishes!

Anika: Thanks so much.

Taylor: Well, my Summer doesn't look half as good as yours, Anika. I have to look for a job, but I'm not really sure where. And as far as my eating goes, I'm not doing so well. My family says I'm relapsing, and my brother was yelling at me and telling me I'm just doing it for the attention.

They just don't seem to understand that it isn't my fault. They make me so freakin mad!

Jillian: It sounds very challenging to be struggling with change and have those closest to you not be understanding. Unfortunately we are unable to choose the dynamics that occur in our family of origin.

Taylor, please try to remember this, you are growing and learning so much about yourself. Sometimes this self growth can be misunderstood or threatening to those around us that are not working through their own difficulties.

Try to offer yourself kindness and know that inside of you (inside all of you) there is a guiding light. Continue to explore and embrace that.

Taylor: Thanks, I guess I need to start seeing my therapist more often now and not skip so many sessions.

Jillian: If that will be helpful, then try that.

There is this quote that may offer you some comfort. My Yoga teacher often says this during difficult poses. "Let yourself fall into the muck. You must go through the sticky stuff to rise up, just as the Lotus Flower does."

Be well, Taylor.

Taylor: I'll try.

Min: I want you all to know I'm going to miss everyone here so much. I really hope I can come back at the end of August to see everyone, but I'm not really sure where I'll be. My parents are thinking about sending me to Summer school because they think it could help me get into a better college.

Taylor: Wow, how can you think about staying in school for the Summer?

Would you go home and see your family in between?

Min: I'm not sure yet. They might plan a trip to come see me if I'm staying somewhere around here.

Carly: Min, is that what you really want, or are you trying to keep them happy?

Min: You know I'm not really sure. I mean, I do want to be able to go to a good college, but I also really want to go home.

Carly: I'm sure you'll be able to get into a good school. You are so smart, and your grades are really good.

Maybe you should just focus on having fun this Summer.

Jillian: Min, I have watched you learn so much at our groups.

I believe you have gained new insights and strength. It is important for you to explore what you most deeply desire and allow it without judgment.

I wish you wonderful moments as you make these transitions.

Min: Thank you for your kindness. It truly means so much to me.

Jillian: You are welcome.

Carly or Stephanie, would either of you like to talk about what things are going like for you?

Carly: I will.

I'm planning to work at a camp for youths with learning disabilities. I've worked there for the last three years. I'm really looking forward to it. I wanted to tell you guys that I found this really great web site called *About Face* where you can send advertisements that are potentially harmful to women, and they'll post them to promote awareness. It even gives addresses of the main advertising companies so you can contact them if you feel like writing a letter directly. I think I'm actually going to write something because I'm so sick of doing nothing.

Stephanie: That sounds really interesting. I'll definitely check it out.

Jillian: Thank you for sharing such a valuable website. What an empowering channel this can be.

Carly, it is wonderful to hear you be so excited about your Summer work. Those children are fortunate to have you spending time with them.

Carly: Thank you. I really cannot wait. It's like I feel peacefulness when I am there – kind of weird, but it's true.

Jillian: Not weird, Carly. You are aware of something that offers you happiness.

Good for you!

Stephanie, would you like to tell us about yourself?

Stephanie: I'm just heading home for the Summer.

My sister is scheduled for heart surgery, so I'm going to help out at home. But I've also decided that I'm going to do something I've never done before – and always wanted to. I'm signed up for a dance class, and although I'm a little nervous about it, I'm really excited.

Jillian: That is exciting! You have learned many new things about yourself over the past weeks and it's taking you to new opportunities. Enjoy each moment!

Stephanie: I will definitely try.

If I could I have something else I want to share with all of you. I'm really proud of it, although it was difficult to write. My therapist was actually the one who suggested writing it, because she felt I was ready.

It's kind of long – are you sure it's Okay?

Jillian: I think the group would love to hear it.

Stephanie reaches into her backpack and takes out an envelope. She opens it and takes out a note written on beautiful violet stationery.

Stephanie: It's a letter to my eating disorder. Here goes:

Dear Eating Disorder,

You have been part of my life for a very long time, and we have come to know one another almost as intimate partners. In fact, you know me so well you can probably predict my thoughts and actions even before me at times. You have been a presence in my life that I unknowingly thought was necessary, no, essential – for such a long time. And you were always there when I thought I needed you. When I felt hollow and invisible – like I fit in nowhere and didn't even belong in my own life – you were there for me.

You helped to bring me the attention and recognition that I so needed. You were my escape from the world when it felt so cold and dismissing. You soothed me by dulling my pain when my sadness became too great. You sheltered me from my fears and my nightmares. And for this, I thank you. But now, dear friend, I think it's time for us to find our separate paths. You see, I think I'm ready to go the distance without you. I have begun a new journey, and on this one, you will not be needed. It's been difficult realizing this – and sad – and I have never been good at separations.

And I must tell you that in deciding whether or not you could come along, I looked long and hard at all our times together. And in all honesty, although you were there for me like no one else, you also took from me that which I so deserved. You were seductive in your ways, and although I thought you helped me, you also made me believe that if I didn't go along with you, I was unworthy – at times even less than human. You had me believing that I had to be perfect in order to be accepted by you and others.

But when I thought I was getting close, you would always raise the bar. You had me believing that I always needed to change to be liked by you and the people around me and that this change involved experiencing pain – both physical and emotional. You know the old saying, "No pain, no gain." Well, I took this too far. It seemed to be our motto at times. You had me believing that girls had to be less than who they really were to be successful. You had me believing that reduction was the only way to happiness.

But what I didn't know, was that there were other answers and ways around this pain. I didn't realize that feelings could be allies or compasses to help me navigate decisions. I didn't realize that there were healthy ways to deal with feelings that seemed overwhelming. I never realized before that within this ever-changing body of hormones there was a little girl inside who was aching to be loved, held, and accepted – one who wanted so badly just to sing, dance, love, laugh…A little girl who had in front of her a whole life, a life in which to do all of these things. I wish that you had told me this. In fact, there are so many things that you never told me.

I never realized before that there were people who loved me just the way I was. I never realized that I could love so deeply and so unconditionally. I never realized before that within my life there could be such promise of dreams… That someday, sometime, another child out there somewhere would be able to look into my eyes and truly understand the power of hope, understanding, and connection.

And so, my friend, it's time to go our separate ways. I wish I could say that I will visit you periodically, but I'm not exactly sure where I'll be. One thing I know for sure is that I will think of you, from time to time, because you are a part of me.

Goodbye for now,

Stephanie

Jillian: Stephanie, what a truly amazing letter. It is difficult for me to find the words to tell you how moving this is.
You are very courageous to write such a letter.

Stephanie: Thank you. It just felt right, and then when I sat to begin it – everything just flowed out of me.

Carly discreetly moves to the floor and sits holding a pillow, while wiping tears from her face.

Jillian: Thank you for sharing this personal, deep relationship with us that you have experienced with your eating disorder.
Excuse me, Carly, are you okay? I see you have moved to the floor with a pillow.

Carly: Yes, I'm fine.
I am just such a sap tonight. I can't believe I am crying.
Your letter, Stephanie, really spoke to me. I cannot thank you enough for bringing it here this evening.

Stephanie: Well, I hope it was helpful. When I saw you crying, I was afraid reading this upset you in some way.

Carly: No. You have helped me more than you may know.

Jillian: It is wonderful to have emotion in this room this evening.

Knowing the connections we have formed, it is natural and healthy for each of you to be struck with various feelings in relation to each other. You began this group together and you will end it together. The bonds between everyone in this room will remain as you continue on your journeys independently.

Anika: Stephanie, I don't know what to say either except, thank you. Thank you for sharing so much of yourself with us.

I have learned so much from the people in this group. I wish we could go on meeting forever. We could share all of each other's milestones and challenges together.

Jillian: I understand it is difficult to think of not being part of each other's lives after sharing so much together. It's even difficult for me.

I feel grateful that all of you have allowed me to become part of your lives.

As we continue our evening together, I would like to have us all partake in an activity that will hopefully be helpful as we part tonight. In planning this activity I believe preparation for change and ceremonies, which mark these rites of passage, can help to ease the anxiety that can sometimes accompany them.

So, as a final exercise or ritual, if you will, I have brought in cloth-covered handmade journals I would like you all to accept as a gift.

For a little while I would like you to take turns writing in each other's books a note of farewell. I also ask that you enclose some thoughts about what you have been given from each person.

After we end our group this evening, I would like to encourage you to stay close to these journals and use them in the same way you would our group.

Anika: Jillian, thank you for this appropriate gift. This will be so helpful for me not only now, but I believe for the rest of my life.

Jillian: Enjoy it!

Carly: Excuse me, even though I cannot believe I am crying about this now, I want all of you beautiful girls to know you will be a part of me forever.

This has been the most encouraging part of my recovery. I love all of you so much.

Jillian: Carly, I think it's wonderful you are embracing your feelings and this experience.

Min: Listening to what you said, Carly, I agree.

Being in America has carried a lot of challenges for me. But this group has surpassed all of the educational experiences I have had. You are all teachers to me. Because of this group I have been able to learn who I really am.

Thank you doesn't feel like it says enough to me.

Jillian: Min, I think you have also been a teacher in our group. I am grateful you allowed yourself to be open to new ideas and ways of thinking.

I wish you great success as you continue to discover about yourself.

Min: Thank you for your kind words.

Stephanie: I would like to offer my deepest thanks to all of you. This has been the only place – besides my therapist – where I have been able to be "weak" at times. I've always been so afraid to let myself be anything but a caretaker to others. I have learned so very much about finally being there for myself. It's like that old airplane saying, "If your plane is having flight issues who do you put the oxygen mask on first – yourself or your child?" Well the answer is yourself because what good are you to others if you don't care for yourself.

Jillian: Stephanie, you have worked very hard here and in your individual therapy.

Have a wonderful time as you continue to discover there is enough nurturing in you to care for yourself while being there for others.

Week Nine: Moving Forward

Stephanie: Thank you.

Taylor, I'm so sorry, I didn't mean to speak before you.

Taylor: Don't' worry about it. It's no big deal. I'm just in this funk and with our last group – I feel crappy.

But I want to say thanks to all of you. This group is probably the truest friends I have ever had.

Thanks for accepting me as I am. I hope you all have great recoveries – you deserve it!

Stephanie: Thank you, Taylor. I have enjoyed getting to know you. I hope you can begin to give yourself more credit – you definitely deserve that!

Taylor: I'm hoping to try.

Jillian: Taylor, I am not sure you recognize the growth you have made here. The first group you weren't sure if you were coming back. You did, and you were greatly committed to each and every one of us.

I hope as you continue with your individual therapist you will be able to finally offer yourself the appreciation you so greatly deserve.

Taylor: That would be nice.

The girls pass their journals around their circle. There is comfortable silence as they intently record their thoughts for each other.

Jillian: Wow, this was a very powerful and meaningful exchange between all of you.

As we prepare to end this evening, I will not be reciting our usual Words of Hope. Because this will be our last official group together, I wanted to offer you all something a little more. I would like to offer all of you **Well-Wishings**.

Let me explain.

The Buddhists have a wonderful practice of saying their prayers, not only to themselves, but aloud. They believe that by recanting these prayers, they are spreading their blessings and offerings to all of mankind. The multi-colored flags that hang outside on the porches of many Buddhist homes are prayer flags. Buddhists believe that when the wind blows, these flags deliver prayers of peace, healing, and protection throughout the world. These prayers are also called Well-Wishing or Offerings.

I have prepared for all of you, my own Well-Wishings, so as each of you move forward in your lives, you can carry with you my blessings. I believe these offerings carry amazing healing energy with them.

Relax, be comfortable, and allow yourselves to take in these compassionate, caring thoughts from me to each of you.

May you find peace within and comfort from the arms of others

May you walk through life uninhibited by the shadows of shame

May you cradle the sanctity of your needs

May you embrace the true magic of your womanhood

May you uncover the opportunities that arise out of unsilenced emotion

May you find contentment in the mere practice of being human

May you dance to life with your entire being

As you dance, may others join in by the power of your example

I believe all of you and your abilities to move on from here.

We will be coming together again August 25 – Tuesday, at six-thirty in the evening in this same space.

I look forward to this time when we will meet again.

Taylor: I was wondering if you all would like to walk out together tonight.

Stephanie: Absolutely!

Week Nine: Moving Forward   207

Carly: I'm in!

Anika: I would enjoy that.

Min: Sure, that would be nice.

Jillian: Be well, all of you. You will be in my thoughts.

The girls exit the room as a group. Jillian smiles and extinguishes the flame on the candle that flickers on the bookshelf.

Coming Back Together

Coming back together is not something I would consider a core struggle, but I do consider it something that can have many differing effects on someone who has been a part of a group.

Coming back together allows for the group members to reunite and gather strength, support, and insight from others they have developed relationships with. Oftentimes, these are individuals who truly understand their struggles. It can be a very powerful experience for many girls working through recovery. With this being said, for some of the girls it may also create or add to the anxiety that they may already feel.

With many of the groups I have facilitated, I have found that the ability to reunite after some time has passed, can be very therapeutic. This type of meeting reflects the true challenges of recovery by allowing the girls to hear and share how experiences of coping skills and new behaviors may be working or not working. It is an opportunity to experience the support that they remember as they experience new supports, connections, or communities, outside of the group that they may or may not have even discovered yet.

Managing Coming Back Together

When a group comes back together after some time, it is imperative to provide the group with a **consolidation of gains**. I have found that in talking about what accomplishments have been made, and highlighting what they may have been able to do, the girls are given a stronger foundation to move forward with. It is a time for me to offer them strength and also reinforce skills to assist them, regardless of where they may be in their process of recovery.

As you read this final Week, through the group members own stories, you may begin to understand that recovery is a process of peaks and troughs. As scary and uncomfortable as this can be, every time you climb a little higher on the mountain of recovery, you are making progress, no matter how many times you may fall. Believe in your own recovery and use the experience of these young women to remind you that recovery from an eating disorder is anything but easy. Yet, it will be worth it someday when you recognize you have a life that is full, happy, and safe, while leaving your eating disorder behind. Trust in yourself and believe in the process. You are capable of prevailing in your recovery!

> It's so funny how we all had this notion we would
> have it all together by the time we meet again.
>
> *– Stephanie*

Jillan: Welcome back. It's so good to see you. I feel so grateful that everyone could make it here this evening with such busy schedules.

Tonight we are gathering one last time, on this balmy late Summer evening. My hope is that in being together again, each of you will be able to anchor yourselves within this supportive and familiar setting you all have worked hard to create. After ending this group a few months ago and venturing out into your lives, it is my intention that coming back to each other will give each of you added strength and courage to continue on in your journeys.

During our time apart, I have reflected on the many body image struggles women in general experience. In exploring this, I was reminded over and over just how strong and powerful these thoughts and feelings can be. I am truly amazed by the endurance you each demonstrate in regards to your recovery. All of you have become a true inspiration for me. For this, I thank each and every one of you.

Anika: It's a bit strange to think that a nurse who facilitates a group is inspired by us.

Jillian: I understand, Anika, how this can seem strange, but I assure you I have learned from everyone in this group. Try to give yourself more credit for all the growth and change you have experienced.

As we begin this evening together, I invite you all to kneel on the floor with me and pick out a handful of these ancient glass beads from this basket, in the middle of our circle. I ask that you keep them close to you as our evening evolves.

*The girls join Jillian on the floor. Lively exchanges occur
as the group examines the basket of beads.*

Min: What beautiful beads. I bet they would make stunning
jewelry.

What are they for?

Jillian: I agree that they are beautiful and I hope you all enjoy
having them with you this evening.

As we experience this evening together the idea behind
these beads will make more sense. For now, please keep them
close to you, enjoying how they feel and look.

I am very eager to hear how all of you are doing. Who
would like to begin?

Carly: I would love to.

It's so great seeing everyone! I missed each of you! So much
has happened.

I don't really know where to begin. Is there a particular way
you want me to do this?

Jillian: You are doing great.

It would be wonderful to know how you're doing and what
your Summer has been like.

Say as much or as little as you want.

Carly: Well, all in all, it's been a pretty amazing Summer, but with
a lot of ups and downs.

I spent most of the Summer working at a camp for kids with
learning disabilities, which was incredible but challenging. The
camp was set up so you would spend most of the time with the
same group. Actually they called it a "pod". And in some ways,
it was great, because you really got to know each other, but if
you didn't get along with everyone, you were kind of stuck.

I became really close to one of the campers in my pod,
a little girl with Tourettes Syndrome, and we were basically
inseparable. There was this amazing connection between us
right from the start and she really trusted me. She really didn't
talk to anyone else. I tried not to favor her so much, but it was

hard because she was made fun of by everyone, even the other counselors. I don't know where they got some of those counselors. And because I was a senior counselor, I was supposed to supervise them. It was really frustrating at times. I'd get so mad by the end of the day.

Sometimes I'd call home and talk with my parents. They tried to be understanding and supportive, but my dad would basically give me the old "I'm sure you'll do the right thing." I guess I just don't understand why people treat each other the way they do. Part of me feels like I'm an adult now, you know? We're not in high school anymore! And I think it's going to be different, no more cattiness or backstabbing. And then I'd get so intolerant of them and so disgusted I'd begin to feel I was no different from them.

Perhaps the reason it was so painful was because I saw how this innocent little girl was so unprotected by life. Maybe I could relate to her – living in a world that can feel so unsafe and judgmental, where you have to be less of yourself to fit in. I found myself really trying not to get depressed, trying to maintain some kind of perspective that the whole world isn't like this. I'd think of you guys, but it was hard not to give in. I hope I don't sound too self righteous and negative.

And then there was my eating. I noticed this pattern. At the end of a really bad day, I'd start berating myself. I'd begin to feel negatively about my body, my skin, or anything else I could find to trash. I'd compare myself to everyone else, and then I'd feel guilty about being so hard on myself. From there, it would just snowball. And it's funny, because although on some levels I knew my eating was fine and I was getting the right amount of exercise, I'd feel compelled to change something. It's so weird how my overall frustration with things I can't control leads to my wanting more control over my body.

It's such a relief to explain this to people I know will understand. I've missed you guys.

I wish we could be part of our own pod and go through our lives together.

Coming Back Together

Stephanie: I would really love that too, Carly.

    The camp sounds like it was really hard for you, but what an amazing experience. It must have been really difficult not to become over-involved with these kids.

    I think you look really great and happy.

Carly: Thanks, Stephanie!

Jillian: Carly, it sounds like this Summer has offered you many opportunities to learn and understand about who you are, what is important to you, and how different situations may cause you to feel.

Carly: I guess I haven't really looked at all of this in that way.

Jillian: Carly, I wonder how this insight about yourself feels to you?

Carly: It's funny you ask me that. Just this morning I was thinking how I feel much more strong and at ease in my life – mainly because of my new ways of coping. Yet, there is this sense of uneasiness that I feel every so often.

    It's like I am on a canoe just floating in the water and I am unsure of what is going to happen. Will a huge wave crash on top of me or will I drift to a wonderful lush land.

    This all feels so uncertain at times.

Jillian: What a wonderful way to express what you have been experiencing.

    It is important to realize the way you were coping and living your life being run by your eating disorder, when we began meeting, offered you a false sense of safety. Now, you have discovered new tools and these shifts that have occurred within you definitely offer you new strength and opportunities. Yet, this can all feel very scary at times. It is new. You have lived with your old way of thinking for many years and feeling comfortable with these changes takes time. Be patient.

    For now, maybe you can just relax and enjoy the calm place you have discovered "being on your raft." Just be.

Carly: Thank you, Jillian. That is very helpful for me. I do have to remember recovery is a process and there is not just one clear cut way that it happens.

Jillian: You're welcome. Who would like to talk next?

Taylor: I don't have much to say, but I'm going to sit on the floor if that's okay – these chairs still get to me.

Taylor appears withdrawn and sad as she moves to sit on the floor.

Jillian: Sure. Like always when we are together, please get as comfortable as possible.

Maybe you can share with us how things have been going for you over the Summer.

Taylor: Not much to share. It's nice to see everyone though, but I feel as though I made a mistake in coming this evening.

I didn't decide until this afternoon I was coming. I mean I don't want to pull everyone else down, because I haven't made much progress with my behaviors. I spent way too much time around my stupid house this Summer and probably too much time thinking. I've been having a lot of weird memories and dreams lately. My mother says if there's no drama in my life I look to create it. I really have been remembering things, and it's kind of freaking me out. I've also been getting a lot of strange sensations in my body when I have these memories.

Actually, I guess they've been going on for a while, because my boyfriend and I broke up at the beginning of July because of all of it. A lot of the body stuff would happen when we were together, and I would end up getting mad at him for no reason. I tried writing about it, but it just seemed to get worse.

Sometimes I wonder if I am just making the whole thing up. When I deliberately try to remember things, the images just fade away.

Taylor gazes down at the floor.

Stephanie: Have you been seeing your therapist lately?

Taylor: No, she's been on vacation, and anyway, I think I need to find someone else, because she's really kind of weird. She

Coming Back Together

doesn't say anything, just sits and looks at me and nods once in a while. And then I end up saying the stupidest things.

Jillian: I am so glad that you decided to come to the group today. Today is not about evaluating all of our successes or challenges of the Summer. It is an opportunity to come together and once again gather strength, support, and insight from people who understand.

However, now does sound like a prime time to reconnect with your old therapist or find a new one you are comfortable with.

Taylor, remember what I was just telling Carly about. Well, the same holds true for you, in fact for all of you. **As you explore new ideas and shifts occur within you, it can be very uncomfortable. Working through all the pain you have protected yourself from for so many years is a difficult process.** This is why it is so important to have a safe place to talk and work through this trauma you may be remembering.

I wonder if you have been able to tell your therapist there are some things in treatment that make you feel uncomfortable?

Taylor: No way, I really don't think I could do that.

Jillian: Maybe think more about it. Remember that those therapy sessions are for you. Use them in the ways you need.

You deserve to have someone who can help you create the safety necessary to do this work.

Taylor: I guess you're right.

Min: How does your boyfriend feel about the fact you're not seeing him?

Taylor: He thought I was acting "different" because of the group. He said my head was being filled with other's thoughts instead of my own. For a while, we'd spend time together, but things just weren't the same. Then, he just stopped calling as much as he used to, and he wouldn't return my calls. I was really hurt and angry for a while, but it's getting easier.

Jillian, what you told me in our last group about my growth

has really stayed with me. I don't think I want to have anything to do with boys for a while.

Anika: I totally understand what you were saying about feeling like you weren't really entitled to come today, Taylor. It's been a crazy Summer with my family, and you won't believe some of these stories.

Do you all remember how I told you I was going on vacation with my aunt and uncle? They rented a lake house in New Hampshire for the Summer, and I was supposed to spend a few weeks with them.

I arrived there thinking it was going to be a relaxing couple of weeks hiking, biking, and bonding with my cousins, only to find out my mother and aunt had this whole thing planned out for me. I was to follow this strict diet and exercise program that they had developed.

Why didn't I see this coming? I should have known better.

It's funny, because it wasn't really obvious at first – kind of subtle – but then when I would get something to eat, my aunt was always close by, and she'd say, "I think it might be a good idea if you had some of this instead," or, "Maybe you should wait a couple of hours before having that." I felt so trapped and powerless. I felt like I was tricked into going to a diet camp for the Summer. They didn't even talk to me about it. What was I supposed to do, take the bus back home to my mother, the person who probably thought this whole thing up to begin with?

I figured out why my aunt is so obsessed with my body size: She's unhappy with her own body, and I never really saw that before. She has more diet books than a bookstore and more exercise equipment than anyone I know. So I've become her project, but she thinks she's doing this to help me and her sister. I couldn't handle the constraints, so I started overeating like crazy, hiding empty wrappers, trying to replace things so she wouldn't notice they were gone. Things kept going downhill. My parents didn't understand why I wasn't losing weight.

Then, I started to totally freak out. I realized I was going to have to start shopping for my internship soon, and I really didn't want to buy a bigger size. I started writing profusely and talking to supportive people online.

My feelings poured out all over the pages. I discovered not only how violated I felt, but I became aware of how scared I was about the internship. I was afraid people wouldn't like me. I was afraid of failing socially, out in the real world, and afraid of being excluded. So what do I do? Alienate myself even more.

As I continued to write, my desire to overeat seemed to lessen. Things seemed more manageable, and slowly they began improving. Now, when I do overeat, it doesn't have the same numbing effect it used to have. It's not an escape anymore. I've discovered escaping is at the core of all of this, my desire to get away from criticism and expectation of everyone else. No wonder being trapped with my family caused such a setback.

I'm getting back on track, and things feel different. It's easier. I don't feel like I'm on a diet or a meal plan. I'm just trying to stay focused on what it is I'm feeling and where I want to go from here.

Jillian: Anika, you have had quite the Summer.

I'm sorry it was such a painful experience for you to be with your aunt and uncle. Yet, you have learned to utilize some really effective coping strategies to help yourself when you're feeling desperate. It is hopeful you were able to find your way back. Your experience truly demonstrates the strength you have developed through all of your struggles.

Anika: Thanks. I do feel stronger.

For the first time I feel like Me!

Jillian: That's wonderful, Anika.

Min or Stephanie: Would either of you like to tell us what has been happening?

Min: I will.

The timing of this group worked out really well for me.

Believe it or not, I start back to school again in a few days, so I decided to come back a day early in order to attend the group. I'm staying with a friend until the dorms officially open. We're planning on going into Boston after this because I've never been there. I'm really excited about it.

I can't believe this Summer is almost over.

Carly: So, whatever happened with Summer school? Did you end up going?

Min: No. Actually, I spent the Summer at home with my family.

It wasn't easy convincing them to let me come home, but ultimately it worked out. My father was the hardest to convince. He interpreted my not wanting to go to school during the Summer as being disrespectful to him. It was difficult for him to understand I just needed a break and I was tired of being away from home. He ultimately left the decision up to me, and I felt so guilty. Neither decision felt right. When I finally made the decision to go home, he was different to me, colder and less available than before. He said I was different – more independent and willful. It was difficult to be there at first, especially after being so homesick for so long, only to have him misunderstand.

Carly: Did your mom understand?

Min: She did understand, but then this caused tension between them. She wanted to be supportive to me, but she also felt a loyalty towards my father.

The other difficult part about being home was being around my friends. They are now all caught up in dieting trends, trying to meet the ideals of the media and a long way from seeing the potential dangers. I guess being here has changed me. It's hard to go home to see some things haven't changed.

I'm much more analytical then I was before. It's harder for me to just accept things as they are

One good thing I've noticed, that has occurred, is my dad is changing – slowly. We've been talking more than we used to.

Coming Back Together

He's beginning to see I'm not just being belligerent for the sake of it, I am just maturing and becoming more independent. Some things just take a while, I guess. He's going to be traveling on business in a few weeks, and he said he'll try to visit for my birthday.

Jillian: Min, it sounds like this Summer has been a time for you to remain true to yourself. You have allowed yourself to have a voice and discover more of who you really are. I think it is wonderful that you were able to pay attention not only to where you needed to be for the Summer, but who it was important for you to relate with.

Thank you for sharing.

Min: You are welcome.

Stephanie: I have to say, I think it's so funny how we all had this notion we would have it all together by the time we met again. I guess that is truly wishful thinking. It seems like life has sent us all challenges since we last were together.

For me, it's been a really hard Summer – not so much in terms of food, just emotionally. I've actually been seeing my therapist twice a week for a while and dance class has been a way for me to stay connected with my body. I will explain.

My sister went in to have her surgery at the beginning of June, and everyone expected she'd have this intense period of recovery but then be much stronger than ever before. She's only nine years old, and she' gone through so much. She's never really been able to be a kid and do the active things kids do. We thought, now that she was older, her body had grown enough to support the surgery. But when they operated on her, they found that the tissues surrounding her heart were unable to sustain the operation. So now they're saying her heart can't be repaired, and her prognosis is poor. She's been at home since then and getting progressively weaker. It's like her body has just stopped fighting because it no longer has the hope of surgery anymore. It's so hard to be with her and know someday she won't be here anymore.

I feel so selfish for thinking about my own problems. When I look at her life, I have no right to be unhappy. And I feel guilty for living, for going on with my life and for getting stronger. I feel like I'm abandoning her – and my mom. I'm so torn, because more than ever before I want my own life. I want to be happy.

Carly: Oh, Stephanie, I am so sorry.

Stephanie: I know, thank you. That means a lot to me.

If I could I would like to share this with all of you. I know it doesn't make much sense, but I have to tell you this.

The other night, I had this really bizarre dream in which my sister and I were connected to some weird looking machine with all these wires. It didn't look like anything I'd ever seen before. It had a pump of some kind, and it was pumping life into me as it was taking it from her. It was so strange. I felt such a sense of sadness and powerlessness. But then, at the very same time, I also had this unexplainable feeling inside that everything would be okay with me. In fact, this will be the first time in ten years I will be starting a new school year feeling moderately Okay about my body and no longer requiring a meal plan.

Jillian: Stephanie, it does sound like a very challenging and painful Summer. I am grateful you were seeing your therapist more often – that was a wonderful way to nurture yourself during this time of uncertainty.

I think your dream is beautiful and demonstrated so much of the inner work you have done.

I am glad you were able to come back here and share all of this with our group.

Stephanie: Me too. Thanks!

Jillian: This has been a powerful evening. I find it so interesting that all of you girls exhibit such responsibility to each other, even after the long Summer break. I wonder if this is due to the strong bond that had formed with all of you earlier this spring,

Coming Back Together

or if it's a reflection of your innate sensitivity. Perhaps both. So attentively you all listen to each other, and how easily you seem to understand each other as each of you spoke of your difficulties and victories. Listening to all of your challenges and triumphs, it is obvious to me this is not just about body image and numbers anymore. Each of you has a meaningful story to be told.

All of you have done your own work in the way it needs to be done just for you. I applaud each of you for your courage, honesty, integrity, and spirit you have demonstrated in our groups together. There is something very powerful about women gathering together that helps promote healing and growth. I would like to encourage all of you to connect with the great strength and guiding light within yourselves. Once you are able to reach this part of yourself, I believe anything can be possible.

I would like all of you to brainstorm with me for a few minutes. As you reflect on your experiences living with an eating disorder, I would like you to think about what you would say or offer to all girls, of all ages, and all cultures. If it helps, try to envision yourselves as the wise elders, sisters, or mentors chosen to bring your gift of hope and wisdom to others.

Since you are sitting next to me, Anika, would you mind starting? Then we will just continue around the circle until it feels complete.

I will write them down as we go along.

Anika: Sure, I will begin.
I would say, be proud of who you are.

Carly: Dance to your own rhythm.

Taylor: Create the balance you crave.

Stephanie: Allow yourself to need.

Min: Surround yourself with people who encourage you to be strong in whom you are.

Anika: Me again, I would say give yourself a voice in your life.

Carly: I wish I was taught this…media messages of TV, radio, internet, and magazines trick you – protect yourself from this game.

Taylor: Look in the mirror and like what you see.
I know it seems stupid but it's all I got right now.

Stephanie: It's great, Taylor.
I would like to say, acknowledge and respect your feelings.

Min: True comfort lies within yourself.

Taylor: Hey, I actually have one more.
Trust yourself.

Jillian: Wow, that was truly uplifting.
As I listen to the wisdom each of you offered, I have this fantasy of preserving your words. In fact, maybe someday I will, with your permission, use your words in a book. Of course your privacy would be protected. I feel you all have such valuable thoughts and insight, that when shared with others can only have a positive effect. In fact, I believe that it would be amazing to utilize each of these thoughts that you all just expressed, to offer support and guidance for many other young women who struggle to move forward in their recovery and for young girls who have not yet begun to turn sideways in the mirror of wonder.

Min: I would be truly honored.

Stephanie: Me too. It would be like a piece of our group would always continue on.

Anika: That's very exciting to think about.

Carly: I think the more people we can help, the better.
I wish I was a part of this group a long time ago!

Taylor: My thoughts might need major editing, but I wouldn't mind.

Jillian: Well, it's quite an idea, but for now I would like to bring

Coming Back Together

our focus back to these last moments we will be sharing as a group.

I would like us all to participate in a closing ceremony, one that will commemorate not only our time together, but one that will symbolize our connectedness. I am asking all of you to do this because I believe that **many of the problems women experience in their lives occur as a result of their feeling isolated – disconnected from themselves and from others.** It is also my belief that it is in the connections we form with others that true healing can occur.

Right now if you would all join me on the floor. Please place the beads you chose earlier and have held close to you throughout the evening back into this basket they came from.

The group sits on the floor in a circle around the basket. Taylor appears disappointed as she places her beads in the basket. The other girls look expectantly towards Jillian.

Taylor: I was hoping to keep these.

Jillian: I promise you will be able to, Taylor, we are not done.
Now, if you would, each of you may choose a new handful of beads from the basket!

One by one, each girl reaches into the basket to collect her handful of beads. A subtle smile appears on Taylor's face.

Anika: They are really beautiful.

Min: They look so calming.

Jillian: Yes, they do.
These beads symbolize the bond that has grown between each of you during our time together.

My intention is for each of you to carry these beads with you as we follow our own paths this evening. You may choose to make a necklace or bracelet or some other creative form with these beads. Whatever you decide may the energy shared between us forever resonate in our beads. They are as unique and beautiful as each of you.

I wish you all a life of health and happiness in your mind, your body, and your heart. Best wishes to all of you.

Carly: Jillian, all of you girls, I will never forget you. I refuse to apologize for crying right now.

I will miss all of you.

Stephanie: Thank you all for allowing me to be weak at times.

Every one of you means something special to me. I love you all.

Min: I am excited and sad.

This has been the best foundation for my life.

Thank you for creating an environment for me to grow and learn. You all are very special to me.

Anika: This group will never be very far from my thoughts. Without all of you, I think I would have gone crazy. It amazes me how meeting once a week for nine weeks could have allowed me to learn healthier ways of living.

For this I feel eternally grateful.

Taylor: You all are the best family I have ever had. I must thank you for showing me what respect and acceptance looks like.

I came here tonight struggling, but after experiencing this evening with all of you, I am leaving with a sense of hope I have never known.

You are the best people. Thank you for accepting me and allowing me into your lives.

Jillian: Thank you, Taylor, Anika, Min, Stephanie, and Carly for sharing your stories with me.

This group has been a true honor for me to facilitate. I do hope our paths will meet again, this would be a blessing, if not, the bonds we have developed in our hearts will remain for all of us.

May each of your voices, from within the journey of eating disorder recovery, be heard by many.

❋

Group: Voices Within the Journey of Eating Disorder Recovery

Reflection

As I reflect on the years of co-facilitating Psychoeducational Eating Disorder groups for young women, many emotions arise. First and foremost, thank you to my dear friend (you know who you are) for being my guide in helping those in recovery and encouraging me to take on this project. Your essence is woven throughout these pages. I would also like to express the deep sense of gratitude that I feel and acknowledge that these experiences have been a true honor and privilege.

As time goes on, I am continuously moved by the ability of many amazing young women to share their pain, despair, challenges, and hope. Being a witness to this on different levels at different times has challenged me in my own personal journey of self growth.

At this moment I would like to offer my deepest appreciation to all of you young women who have allowed me into your lives during your recovery. This book is a reflection of the wonderful parts that exist in each and every one of you. Through sharing your struggles and revealing your inner strengths, it has been possible to now offer, so many others who struggle, a glimpse of hope and faith. You are all an inspiration.

In conclusion, I would like to offer this final thought to all women young and old, near and far, who may be struggling with an eating disorder or dealing with body image issues.

May the voices from beyond recovery carry you as you embark and continue on your own personal journey. I wish you strength, understanding, and empowerment.

– Be Well

Annette Aberdale-Kendra

References

Week One

Spiegal, D. and Classen, K. *Group Therapy for Cancer Patients: A Research-based Handbook of Psychosocial Care.* New York, NY. Basic Books, 2000

Lobue, A. and Marcus, M. *The Don't Diet, Live-It Workbook.* Carlsbad, CA. Gurze Books, 1999.

Week Two

Lobue, A. and Marcus, M. *The Don't Diet, Live-It Workbook.* Carlsbad, CA. Gurze Books, 1999.

Brach, T. *Radical Acceptance.* New York, NY. Bantam Dell, 2003.

Keys, A. *The Biology of Starvation.* University of Minnesota Press, 1950.

Week Three

Liu, A. *Gaining.* New York, NY. Warner Books, 2007.

Domar, A. and Dreher, H. *Self-Nurture. Learning to Care for Yourself As Effectively as You Care for Everyone Else.* New York, NY. Penguin Books, 2001.

Lobue, A. and Marcus, M. *The Don't Diet, Live-It Workbook.* Carlsbad, CA. Gurze Books, 1999.

Week Four

Liu, A. *Gaining.* New York, NY. Warner Books, 2007.

Hopps, N. *Relax – Quick!: Simple, Effective Relaxation Processes You Can Do in Moments Anytime, Anywhere.* Eugene, OR. Synergistic Systems, 1995.

Thornton, M. *Meditation in a New York Minute: Super Calm for the Super Busy.* Boulder, CO. Sounds True, 2006.

Week Five

Bourne, E. *The Anxiety and Phobia Workbook.* Oakland, CA. New Harbinger Publication, 2000.

Week Seven

Roth, G. *Feeding the Hungry Heart.* New York, NY. Macmillan Publishing Company, 1982.

Pipher, M. *Reviving Ophelia.* New York, NY. Ballantine Books, 1994.

Gilligan, C. *In a Different Voice.* Cambridge, MA. Harvard University Press, 1982.

Week Eight

Taffel, R. *The Second Family.* New York, NY. St. Martin's Press, 2001.

Nasser, M., Katzman, M., and Gordon, R. *Eating Disorders and Cultures In Transition.* New York, NY. Taylor and Francis Inc., 2001.

Gilligan, C. and Wilson, M. *Girls Seen and Heard: 52 Life Lessons for Our Daughters.* New York, . NY. Penguin Putnam Inc., 1998.

Week Nine

Borysenko, J. *The Biology, Psychology, and Spirituality of the Feminine Life Cycle.* New York, NY. Riverhead Books, 1996.

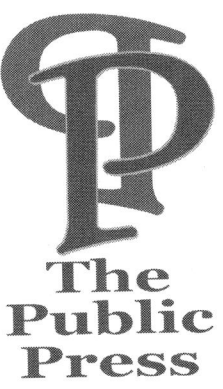

Promoting Free Speech Word-by-Word

The Public Press employs new technologies and the economics of scale – "small" scale, that is – to publish books that might not otherwise see the light of day. We then offer our titles a home so that they are accessible via traditional book trade channels.

The Public Press

We specialize in Author's Editions

For many, an Author's Edition will be the fastest and most reasonable route to publication. With our assistance the author manages pre-press operations, thereby achieving maximum control and financial opportunity at the lowest risk.

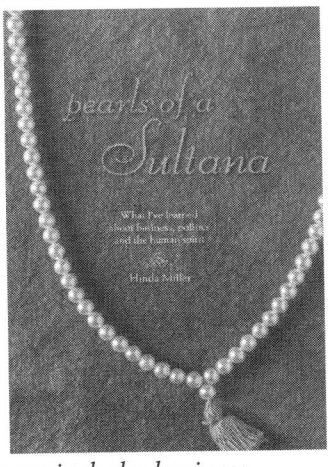

Pearls of a Sultana by Hinda Miller

A memoir of Hinda Miller's experience includes business, politics, spirituality, and more. Drawing from her father's wisdom, Ms. Miller and a partner develop the Jogbra, the original sports bra, and grow their company into a women's sportswear powerhouse they sell to a corporate giant. After her career as an executive, she embarks on a new career as a Vermont State Senator. Throughout all her ventures, Hinda Miller is guided and anchored by a strong connection to the practice of yoga. The book documents her preparation for a new venture as a Sultana, a woman of experience and wisdom who is always practicing, always learning, and always grateful.

℗ The Public Press

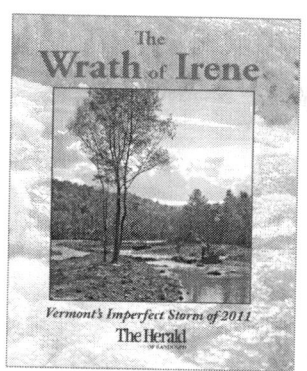

We specialize in *Community Supported Books (CSBs)*

Some books have as their primary goal to support a specific community. Inspired by Community Supported Agriculture (CSAs) Community Supported Books can reach special interest markets that are not served by commercial publishers.

Books by Stephen Morris:

Stripah Love

While our hero (Artie) has achieved success, it's summarily withdrawn from him, arbitrarily, and unfairly. The lady of our tale, Shea, has achieved success, only to find that it exists in close proximity to the law of the jungle. Set on the muddy clam flats of Massachusetts Bay, this is a love story about fish and a fish story about love.

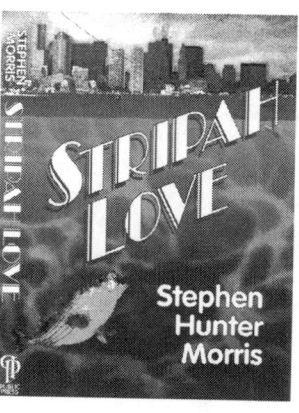

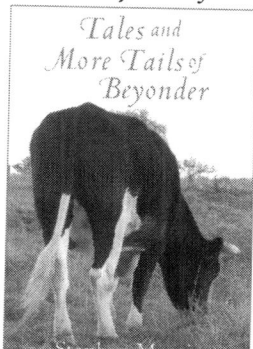

Tales (and More Tails) of Beyonder

Stephen Morris is an indefatigable chronicler of life in Beyonder, and this is his best work. This is a collection of his shorter pieces. His offerings on Mud Season and Vermont Holidays are particularly memorable.

Stephen Morris's *Vermont Trilogy*

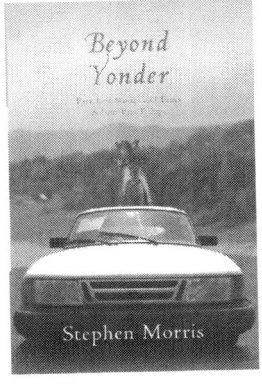

Beyond Yonder

When Darwin Hunter decides to update Over Yonder Hill (Alton Blanchard's history of the tiny Vermont hamlet of Upper Granville), the result is Beyond Yonder, a chronicle of the cultural divide between the entrenched natives and the invaders from the Land of Flat. From "Babysitters" to "Zucchinis" the contrasting world views are examined and skewered.

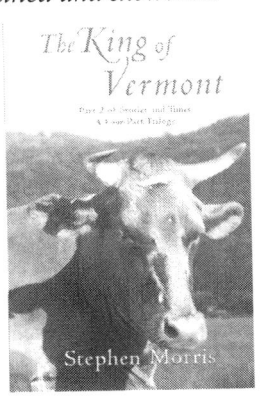

The King of Vermont

A chance comment on Vermont's most popular talk show, Straddlin' the Fence, lands Darwin Hunter in a three-way race to be elected State Senator. Set against a political landscape as rocky and muddy as the garden during Mud Season, Darwin combats his wily, experienced opponents with his only long suit–the truth.

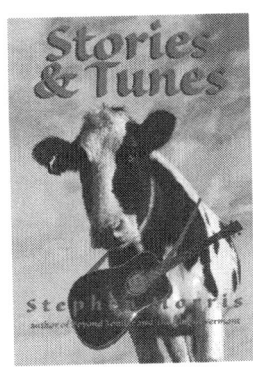

Stories & Tunes

The long-anticipated third volume of Morris's Vermont trilogy. Darwin Hunter is now the MegaBucks Czar, a man with unassailable authority over the state lottery. After an epiphany that reveals to him the regressive nature of this institutionalized gambling, Darwin becomes a modern day Robin Hood, using his power to more fairly distribute the wealth, at least in the Brigadoon that is Vermont.

All titles by Stephen Morris $12.95
(plus $3 shipping and handling) from The Public Press
100 Gilead Brook Road, Randolph, VT 05060
(802) 234.9101 ThePublicPress.com

Made in the USA
Charleston, SC
11 September 2012